Alice Pelton is one of the world's leading experts on women's experiences with contraception and reproductive health. Since founding The Lowdown in 2019, she has become a key spokesperson for driving change in women's health. Alice has collaborated with the UK government on women's health policy and is frequently asked to comment on women's health issues by media outlets, including Channel 4, Radio 4 *Woman's Hour*, *The Times*, *Daily Mail*, *Vice* and *Wired* magazine.

At The Lowdown, Alice works closely with medical directors Dr Melanie Davis-Hall and Dr Frances Yarlett, GPs who have conducted thousands of one-on-one consultations with women through The Lowdown and in their NHS roles. Together their work has provided invaluable insights into the real-life challenges women face with contraception and reproductive health. These conversations have shaped The Lowdown's content, ensuring it reflects the voices and needs of women. Dr Davis-Hall and Dr Yarlett write or review all of the curated content on the platform and social channels, translating complex medical jargon into relatable, accessible information to help women make informed decisions about their health.

# CONTRACEPTION

**Your essential guide to separating the myths from the medicine**

ALICE PELTON,
DR FRANCES YARLETT &
DR MELANIE DAVIS-HALL

PIATKUS

PIATKUS

First published in Great Britain in 2025 by Piatkus

1 3 5 7 9 10 8 6 4 2



A CIP catalogue record for this book
is available from the British Library.

ISBN: 978-0-34944-151-1 (hardback)
978-0-34944-149-8 (paperback)

Typeset in Sabon by M Rules
Printed and bound in Great Britain by Clays Ltd, Elcograf S.p.A.

Papers used by Piatkus are from well-managed forests
and other responsible sources.

FSC
www.fsc.org
MIX
Paper | Supporting responsible forestry
FSC® C104740

Piatkus
An imprint of
Little, Brown Book Group
Carmelite House
50 Victoria Embankment
London EC4Y 0DZ

The authorised representative
in the EEA is
Hachette Ireland
8 Castlecourt Centre
Dublin 15, D15 XTP3, Ireland
(email: info@hbgi.ie)

An Hachette UK Company
www.hachette.co.uk

www.littlebrown.co.uk

This book is dedicated to any woman or person who has navigated the challenges of hormones, side effects or reproductive health issues. As The Lowdown shows, you are absolutely not alone.

# Contents

# Introduction
## from Alice, Founder & CEO of The Lowdown

### My story

'What on *earth* is wrong with you?' sighs my mother, while I pack up the car. It's 2007, and my eyes are pricked with tears for the third time in twenty-four hours. We've been arguing all morning as I've got my things ready to drive back to university in London. I've been feeling tearful and very irritable; a familiar feeling throughout my teens.

'It's your pill, isn't it?'

I will never forget my mum's words that morning. At that moment, the penny dropped. I had just started taking the combined pill again after getting into a new relationship, and within a couple of days, I felt like I was sixteen again.

I was always known as a 'hormonal' and 'moody' teenager but, looking back now, I wonder how much of this was me and how much was the impact hormonal contraception had on me. Teenage years are such a formative time, when many of us are navigating what our 'normal' even is. During my late teens, I felt that I didn't have a grip on my emotions and could easily roll into a tidal wave of anger and upset, with a lump in my throat and a wobbly voice. Feeling out of control like that is horrible, socially isolating and, frankly, a bit embarrassing.

Until that morning, even my mum, a doctor and psychiatrist, had never linked my mood changes with contraception. But after she did, it sparked a ten-year journey of investigation and personal research in order to try to find a contraceptive that worked for me. I must have tried over seven different methods, but I never seemed to find one that suited me. Every time I got into a new relationship I'd go back to my doctor and try something else, hoping it would click this time. But, yet again, I would struggle to get used to it, suffering with incredible mood swings and being sent on a physical and mental rollercoaster.

Navigating this was no easy task – I had so many questions about my contraception but struggled to find answers. My GP visits barely scratched the surface of my search for information; either there wasn't enough time in the short appointment or they didn't have the expertise or data to answer my questions: 'What's the difference between all of these types of combined pill? And if I don't get on with this pill, which brand should I try next?' Then there were the long waits in a sexual health clinic – where I'd be handed tired leaflets on my contraceptive options that looked like they'd been published before I was even born, only to be told there was a lengthy waiting list to get a coil fitted.

Along the way, I had a long and convoluted process to be diagnosed with endometriosis, a common condition which causes painful periods and made having sex uncomfortable. By the time I hit my thirties, I wanted to start trying for a baby, and this was yet another rollercoaster with even higher stakes for my physical and mental health, including months of trying and an ectopic pregnancy.

It's been a journey! One where I haven't felt listened to and have struggled to find the answers I needed at the time I needed them most. My overriding feeling was: this is not good enough. I have realised first-hand just how broken reproductive healthcare is for women, and that has made me determined to do something to change it. It was only once I started reaching out to other women that I realised so many were having similar experiences. It wasn't me, it was the system.

## What's going wrong?

As I muddled through those years of contraceptive ups and downs, I felt increasingly frustrated by the lack of structured and actionable data on the side effects, symptoms, solutions and reality of using these products. It surprised me that there's never been an accessible place to collect real-life feedback data from women on contraception, at scale. You either spoke to friends, read an intimidating internet forum, or asked your doctor. All of these are small sample sizes, and you're never sure whether one person's experience is the norm or the exception. On top of this, there was no easy way to combine this anecdotal data with the clinical research on contraceptive side effects, symptoms or benefits in a way that a layperson like me could easily understand.

## Bring on the innovation

The more I started delving into the world of contraception and women's health, the more I learnt about what an archaic and underinvested space it is. One of the major underlying problems is that the contraceptive methods we have available to us simply aren't good enough. One study looking at women in the US found that 46 per cent of women had stopped a method of contraception because they were unsatisfied with it,[1] and in another study, concern about side effects[2] was the number one reason why Western women changed from the contraceptive pill.

The poor product choice is in the main part due to the fact that the pharmaceutical industry invests a disproportionately small amount of time and money into developing new ways to stop people getting pregnant. In general, big pharma spends 20 per cent of its revenue from sales of a drug on research and development (R&D), but when it comes to the contraceptive space, just 2 per cent goes on R&D and products.[3] The reasons behind this lack of innovation are complicated – but from what I've learnt, it's a combination of factors mostly linked to money:

- Contraceptives are expensive and difficult to develop, trial and get regulated. It's a risky business giving a healthy person a drug that could result in pregnancy (which is actually, as we explain in this book, one of the riskiest things your body can go through).
- Pharmaceutical companies will never be able to sell contraceptives at the same price as other drugs, such as life-saving cancer medication. In 2018, drug sales for cancer medication were a whopping ten times that of hormonal contraceptives.[4]
- Pharmaceutical companies are also scared about getting sued; there were lots of legal disputes involving contraceptives in the 1980s and '90s, and the PR fallout from these can be damaging.
- Some pharmaceutical companies have (fairly unfounded) fears that any new male methods will erode the established female contraceptive market.

- There's a general perception that we have 'enough' options, and because they are effective at preventing pregnancy, we don't need to invest in any new methods.

## Bring on the expertise

Compounding this problem is the fact that getting good medical advice on contraception and sexual health in many parts of the world is really difficult.

Firstly, as many topics in this book show, explaining the risks and side effects, which are complicated and often subjective issues, inevitably takes time to unpack and explain. I have no idea how a GP or practice nurse can fit a proper contraception consultation into a ten-minute appointment. There are so many questions and options to run through, so it's no surprise that a third of us don't feel we have time during an appointment to discuss everything we want to with a doctor.[5]

Then, there's a lack of medical training. GPs are fantastic holistic practitioners and well suited to counselling on contraception, but many of them don't receive in-depth training in contraception – or in menopause, for that matter – as part of their standard training. Any further training is the GP's choice and may have a personal cost to them upwards of £1,000. This lack of training or focus partly stems from the fact that contraception is, ironically, a fairly unsexy part of medicine, and historically not a part of medicine at all; at the start of the twentieth century, medical students were not taught about birth control.[6] It has taken a long time for sexual and reproductive healthcare to become a medical speciality, and even then, it struggles to compete with the more competitive parts of medicine like cardiology and surgery.

## Bring on the access

Finally, we know that pretty much everywhere in the world, contraception is too hard to access, and for many, trying not to get pregnant is harder than getting pregnant. This ranges from not finding the contraceptive pill brand you want available in your local pharmacy to waiting months for an appointment to get your IUD fitted. The UK has systematically cut funding for sexual health services over the last ten years;[7] in the US the situation is worse, with around nineteen million people lacking reasonable access to contraception.[8]

## The birth of The Lowdown and what we do

Moaning to my boyfriend Keiran about this minefield over dinner one evening, an idea popped into my head. What if we were to gather women's experiences with different methods of contraception at scale, would it be helpful? Would it tell us new or insightful things? Could it help the one billion people worldwide who use contraception to find something that works for them?

To test my idea I created a survey about experiences with contraception, and sent it out to around twenty of my female friends. Within two weeks, I had 500 responses. This level of interest, along with the survey data, confirmed what I now know so well: that millions of women experience side effects from their contraception, that information about this is woefully lacking and that women deserve better.

Armed with the survey results, I set about building the first version of The Lowdown's website as a side project in 2018. Within a year, the website had over 30,000 users a month. I quit my corporate job and decided to work on it full time.

Around the same time, the media attention about women's health started to grow; it felt like every millennial features-writer had woken up to the fact that contraception and reproductive healthcare is broken, and they were contacting me and my team for comment.

The Lowdown has grown into a research platform for women's health that reaches over ten million women a year. We help women get clear, credible and reassuring answers to their health questions in a timely way. We do this by combining thousands of real-life reviews and experiences on products and conditions with content and tools that help women break down and understand the clinical evidence.

If you had told me seven years ago that I would be on telly chatting to Davina McCall about contraceptive side effects, I don't know if I would have believed you. It's taken a lot of PowerPoint pitch presentations to rooms full of (often male) investors, and speaking to anyone who will listen to us, both in person and online, to get to this point. What started as a one-woman mission has grown into a small but tenacious team of people, and it's not lost on me that we're able to fill a whole book – and then some – with everything we've learnt from speaking directly to women since 2018.

I'm proud of the fact that because of The Lowdown, we're finally having a nuanced conversation about contraception, and women are more aware of the side effects, benefits and risks. We're educating women on how to make better contraceptive decisions with world-first tools such as our contraception recommender, an algorithm that shares a personal recommendation based on previous experiences and medical history.

In 2023 we started to expand The Lowdown into a wider research platform for women's health, allowing people to share their experiences with fertility, polycystic ovary syndrome (PCOS), endometriosis, menopause and HRT, some of which are shared in this book. What I've learnt since setting up The Lowdown is that contraception is a gateway to a whole bunch of women's reproductive health topics and conditions because it can be used as a treatment to manage conditions and sometimes mask symptoms. And in all of these areas we have the same set of problems: a system that isn't built with our needs in mind, a lack of data and clinical research, and an overwhelming urge from many women to feel heard.

Tackling these issues and pushing for change is therefore at the heart of what we do. We partner with the NHS to share our insights into women's health so we can improve the status quo. We work with innovators in women's health, to gather anonymised insights on what women really want when it comes to their health, so they can meet our unmet needs. We also work with companies and academic researchers that help to recruit patients for clinical trials, to help increase the number of women that are involved in health research and development, as we are woefully under-represented. Women make up just 22 per cent of phase 1 clinical trial participants,[9] and often reproductive-aged women are excluded from trials in case their menstrual cycle or contraception 'interferes' with the results. Yep, this means most medical treatments have only really been studied on men. If you'd like to get involved in research, Chapter 12 tells you how.

## Using this book

It's no longer just me trying to change the conversation around contraception. This book has been written by myself and The Lowdown's Medical Directors, Dr Melanie Davis-Hall and Dr Frances Yarlett. It's based on the main topics and questions that we have been asked about contraception by thousands of women over the years.

Throughout the book we share data and experiences from women gathered on our review platform and in surveys that we have conducted. We hope to bring to life many of the topics and themes we address, and provide the personal insight that women love about The Lowdown website. This anecdotal data is combined with clinical research, and you will see all of our sources clearly referenced in the endnotes. We also reached out to some of the experts and friends we've made along the way, to get their thoughts on some of the conditions and topics we unpack.

Unlike some books on women's health that fill knowledge gaps with 'woo-woo', something we're good at at The Lowdown as a team is sometimes saying 'we don't know'. So much of this space is under-researched, to the extent that there simply is no clinical research, or no good-enough clinical research, to point you towards. What we can tell you is what doctors and other experts currently think and what thousands of women have told us they've experienced, so you can advocate for yourself until you have found something that suits you – or found answers to your questions about your health.

We would love this book to be a companion that sees you or your friends and family through the key stages of their reproductive life; a book that can be read from cover to cover, or picked up when you feel rusty on a certain topic or method. I especially hope this book can be given as a gift from parents to teenage daughters, or shared between younger women, so they don't have to go through what I did. This book doesn't push one form of contraception over another – there is no 'best' method, because we are all unique in how we experience contraceptives, both hormonal and non-hormonal. While the information we offer isn't a substitute for medical advice, it should ensure you are well informed to make the most of the conversations with your doctor, nurse or pharmacist.

As well as giving practical evidence-based information, I'm keen for this book to offer reassurance and hope. One of the reasons I set up The Lowdown was because I wanted to do something that would help women *right now* – data and content that helps us make the best of the options we currently have. And there are reasons to be optimistic about what's to come – in Chapter 12, we explore how we're five to ten years away from new, improved methods for most men and women. A better contraceptive future is coming our way.

Alice and The Lowdown team
2025

## A note on inclusion

We're proud to be a groundbreaking women's health platform, and while we use the word woman in this book and across our media, we support all people who use contraception. This book is an inclusive sexual health resource for women, trans men and non-binary folk. Statistics and studies referenced in this book may draw on women/female exclusivity because they only featured cisgender female participants. In order for medical research to be more encompassing and inclusive, research should increasingly draw on a diverse range of participants, rather than cisgender people only. This will really help medical advancements and healthcare for all.

# 1

# Not just the basics (but also . . . the basics)

If your secondary-school sex ed consisted of some slides of what sexually transmitted infections (STIs) look like, and the school nurse showing you how to put a condom on, you wouldn't be the only one. While school sex ed might have made you cringe, what's happened – or not happened – in the wider world of health research has likely led to the limited education many of us got as young teens.

Women's health is an area that has been woefully neglected and under-researched across the world (thanks, patriarchy). In 2022, 2.4 per cent of publicly funded research in the UK was dedicated to reproductive health[1] (in spite of one in three women experiencing a reproductive health or gynaecological condition).[2] Unfortunately, it's no surprise there has historically been a trickle-down effect on the sex education offered to young people. It wasn't until 1993 that it was mandated that women were to be included in medical trials. Is it any wonder that there are still social taboos around things like periods and breastfeeding, when there's a glaring scientific knowledge gap throughout most of history? The 'ha ha, gotcha' element of countless social media videos of men trying and failing to point out the clitoris on a diagram – the part of the vulva that's responsible for the majority of our orgasms – starts to seem less funny.

Thankfully, the tide is turning with campaigners like Bloody Good Period, Irise International and Wellbeing of Women demanding better awareness of menstrual health, equal rights and access to healthcare. But in the grand scheme of things, we're still in the early stages of research for so many conditions, like endometriosis, that can have a debilitating effect on our bodies. Evidence for a genetic basis for endometriosis was only discovered in 2023.[3]

Before we get into contraception in all its forms, and how it can impact your hormones, periods, skin, mood and sex drive – to name a few – we need to look at how the menstrual cycle works. Even if your school days are long behind you and you're muddling through the realities of adulthood, knowing the basics is the key to understanding your body and figuring out which contraceptive might work best for you, both now and in the future as your needs change. Scattered throughout this chapter are common myths which our doctors are often asked about by patients. These were the 'facts' you may have been led to believe during puberty, or ones you've heard in conversation that went accepted, but not fact-checked. Let's get into it.

## The menstrual cycle 101

The menstrual cycle is the process your body goes through to shed the uterus lining every month, which sounds a bit brutal on paper. The average age to get your first period is twelve, and between then and menopause, the average female will have around 450 periods before menopause, or fewer if, for example, you're using hormonal contraceptives or have any pregnancies.[4] While a lot of us start our periods in our early teens, your cycle may not actually become regular for a few years, until around the ages of sixteen to eighteen.[5]

The key to understanding your menstrual cycle is to recognise the different phases, how fertile you are (i.e. likely to get pregnant) in each of them, and how they can make you feel. First up, the basics:

**Phase 1** Follicular phase (i.e., before ovulation): this starts with the first day of your period. The ovaries are getting ready to release an egg and after initially shedding as your period, the uterus lining starts to prepare by becoming thick enough to receive a fertilised egg.

**Phase 2** Ovulation (when the release of an egg from the ovary occurs): typically, people tend to ovulate mid-cycle, about ten to sixteen days before your next period starts. This is when you're at your most fertile. However, the ovulation day varies between individuals and some people may not ovulate in every cycle (read page 26 for more on cycle tracking).

**Phase 3** Luteal phase (after ovulation): the thick uterus lining is maintained ready for a fertilised egg to implant (which means the egg will bury itself in the thick lining), and if it doesn't, then this leads to your period. (The first day of your period is then day one of your new cycle, signalling the start of a new follicular phase.)

How you feel during the phases of the cycle can very much vary person to person and even between cycles. The upcoming info is a general overview that doesn't take into account how the cycle can be affected by specific medical conditions or by taking hormonal contraception (don't worry, though, we'll get to all that in Chapter 5). Before we go into more detail on how each of these stages can make you feel, and what kinds of symptoms you might notice, you should know more about the hormones that are responsible for all of it.

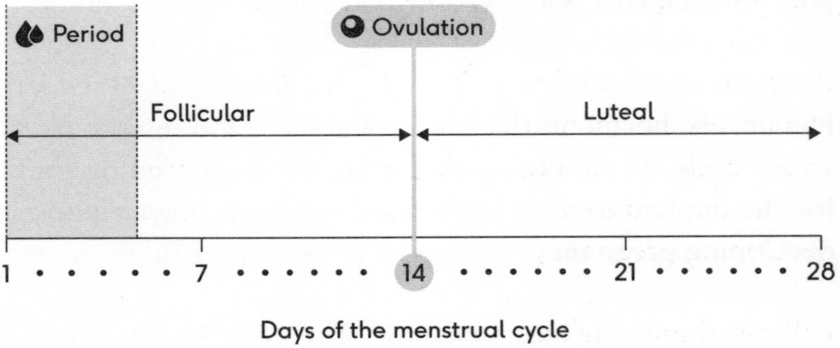


## The hormones at the helm of the menstrual cycle

When we say, 'It must be my period' as an explanation for things like mood swings, irritability or whatever else, we can forget to celebrate how incredible the menstrual cycle is. Your body has the fascinating ability to go through changes every month, all due to the force at the control box: your hormones. Hormones are chemicals that tell the body to behave in certain ways. From the sex hormones that control your menstrual cycle to those that regulate your blood pressure, metabolism and sleep, hormones are created and released by the endocrine system (a network of glands and organs) in our bodies, and are a vital factor in our health. Hormones naturally fluctuate not just over the course of the month, but at key times of change in our lives, like puberty or perimenopause.

The VIPs of the reproductive hormones, which will be popping up throughout this book, are:

**Oestrogen** This helps regulate the menstrual cycle, thickens the uterus lining and enables ovulation. It's the hormone that's responsible for the milestones of female reproductive development during puberty. Oestrogen also has positive effects on your bone, heart and blood vessel health alongside wide-ranging effects all over the body.

**Progesterone** Along with oestrogen, this is the other key female sex hormone that controls and regulates the menstrual cycle. It maintains the lining of the uterus to allow for the implantation of a fertilised egg and then supports a developing pregnancy.

**Follicle-stimulating hormone** (FSH) This is a hormone released from the pituitary gland at the base of the brain. The pituitary gland is a small, yet mighty, organ; it's like the conductor of your body's intricate endocrine orchestra, releasing many of the hormones which dictate how your body functions. When released, FSH stimulates your ovaries to mature eggs, ready for them to be released.

**Luteinising hormone** (LH) Like FSH, LH is produced by the pituitary gland and causes your ovaries to release an egg, which is called ovulation.

Let's look at how these hormones interact when you menstruate (i.e. have your period, if you're not on hormonal contraception) and how these interactions change throughout the cycle. They play a massive role in how you can feel, affecting mood and energy levels (which is why you may want to work *with* your cycle and not against it). It's not clear why some suffer more than others at specific points during their cycle, but it's thought to be related to changing levels of hormones (and possibly serotonin, a chemical that transmits messages between the nerve cells in your brain and body) between ovulation and the start of the next period. Most women experience some discomfort in the days leading up to their period; however, around 5–8 per cent suffer from severe premenstrual syndrome (PMS, page 110) that can disrupt their daily lives.[6]

### Phase 1: Follicular phase, before ovulation

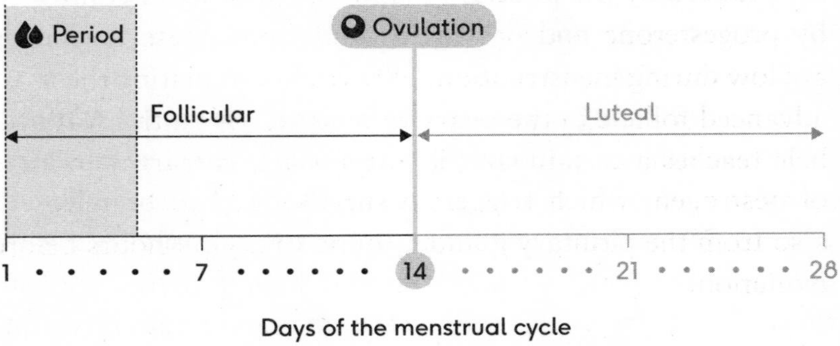


• **WTF is happening?** The follicular phase kicks off with the start of your period, and the first day of bleeding is considered day one of your menstrual cycle. Blood and tissue come from the break-up of the inner lining of the uterus and for most, bleeding lasts between two and seven days. On average, you lose around one to five tablespoons of blood per cycle, which is around 20–90 ml. If that still feels too abstract, that's about one to two shot glasses. The length of time your period lasts, along with the amount of blood loss, varies between individuals, with some having light periods and others bleeding more heavily, so it's helpful to get to know what's normal for you (see page 103 to help work out if your period is normal or heavy).

• **The hormone check-in** Both progesterone and oestrogen are low at the start of this phase and increase as the days progress. When oestrogen is detected in the endometrium (the inner lining of the uterus), it is stimulated to grow and thicken. Oestrogen is mainly produced in the ovaries, though its production is controlled by the release of other hormones made in the pituitary gland. This stage is key for the development of follicles. A follicle is a tiny bag of fluid within the ovary. Each follicle contains just one egg, which it stores until it's mature. In the ten to twenty days before ovulation, FSH is produced by the pituitary gland. FSH release is controlled by progesterone and oestrogen, and when these hormones are low during menstruation, FSH rises, stimulating the most advanced follicle in the ovary to mature. When this VIP follicle reaches a certain size, it starts to release large amounts of oestrogen, which triggers a surge of LH to be released, also from the pituitary gland, around thirty-six hours before ovulation.

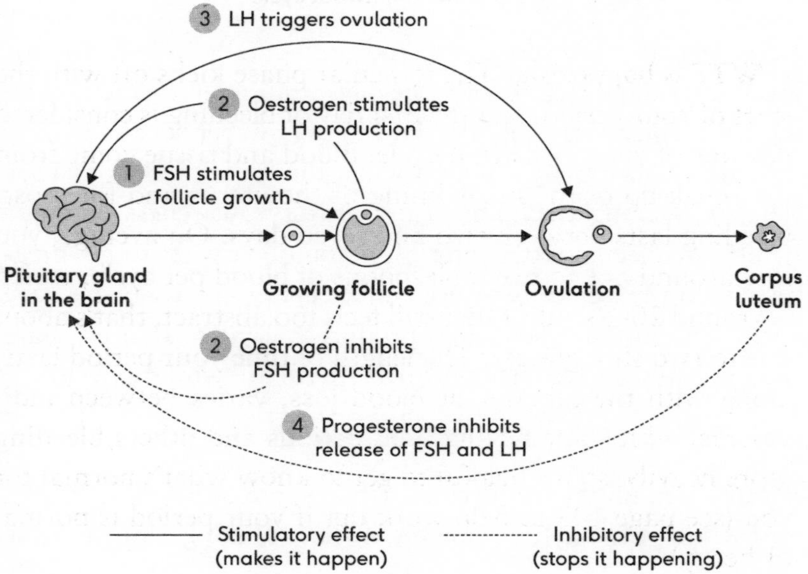

• **How fertile are you?** You are fertile in the days leading up to ovulation – this is called your fertile window. This means that unprotected penis-in-vagina sex in the days before ovulation can potentially result in pregnancy. This is because after sex sperm stays lurking around, ready for the egg to show up. The human body has some ingenious ways to ensure the survival of our species. And one of the admittedly weirder ones is the existence of cervical crypts (aka sperm crypts). These glands are side channels of the cervix (the neck of your uterus) which can store sperm for up to five days (survival rates of the sperm depend on certain conditions, such as the stage of the menstrual cycle). Mucus produced by your cervix works alongside the crypts to protect the sperm until an egg is released during ovulation. Understanding the storage capacity of your cervix may shed a whole new light on your fertile window, and often comes as a surprise to many. Basically, sperm is sneaky.

---

**Q:** Can I actually get pregnant at all times?

**A:** Technically no, you can't! You are actually only fertile for around six days each month (the days leading up to and including when you ovulate and the day after); however, it can be really difficult to accurately pinpoint when this is. So, unless you are reliably tracking ovulation using fertility awareness methods (which we discuss in Chapter 3), if you don't want to get pregnant then the advice is to use contraception anytime you have sex. Men, on the other hand, produce sperm constantly so are theoretically always fertile (if their sperm are working well).

---

• **How you might feel** Periods affect some more than others, and while you may be rejoicing in the amazing natural force that is your menstrual cycle (or the fact that you're not pregnant), you could be struggling with pain, cramps and fatigue. For some, the catalogue of symptoms from your changing hormones feels worse in the days leading up to your period (i.e. premenstrual syndrome, aka PMS), and mercifully gets better the day bleeding starts, or within a couple of days.

• **Your to-do (or not-do) list** Menstrual leave from work is slowly being introduced in some parts of the world – Spain really has their priorities in order[7] – but sadly this isn't feasible for a lot of us. We recommend stocking up on your preferred period products and keeping a stash in all the usual places you might get caught out. If you want to use painkillers, for those with heavy bleeding, anti-inflammatories like ibuprofen can also reduce blood loss by 25–35 per cent.[8] Or, try out heat patches or a TENS (transcutaneous electrical nerve stimulation) machine for portable period pain relief that easily sits under your clothes. Gentle exercise, getting some fresh air, keeping warm and wearing cosy, loose-fitting clothes can help if you are bloated. Your body needs iron to replace lost blood cells and is great at replenishing iron stores from your diet, so you may want to increase your intake of iron-rich foods and eat these alongside foods containing vitamin C, which help iron absorption.

If you really struggle with your period each month, and find that you need to take time off work or can't manage getting out of bed, please speak to your GP. They will investigate possible underlying causes and work on a plan to help relieve or manage your symptoms. While some women may suffer from severe symptoms, it's not normal and you shouldn't have to put up with it. In the Resources section at the back, we've listed some organisations who provide great support around menstrual health.

### Phase 2: Ovulation

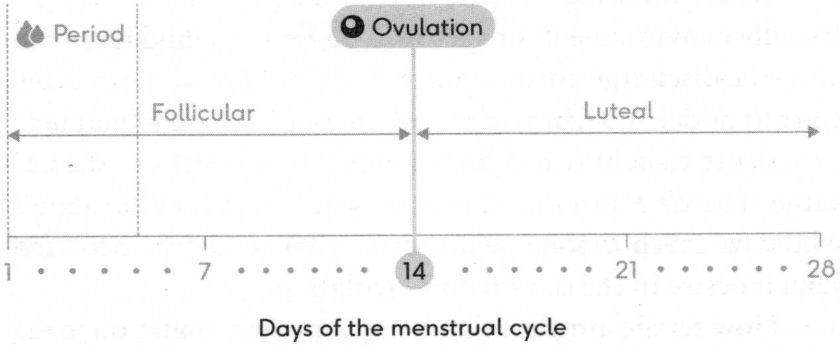


• **WTF is happening?** Ovulation typically occurs mid-cycle, but normally anywhere between ten to sixteen days before your next period (though it varies, both from person to person and sometimes between cycles, too). It's when the follicle breaks open and releases the mature egg into the fallopian tube (the tube that carries the egg between the ovary and the uterus). Some women can experience pain or spotting (light bleeding from the vagina) when this happens. If you do have spotting between periods, this should always be checked by a healthcare professional. A new follicle needs around 120 days to reach maturity, but while many follicles begin this process, usually just one makes it to full maturity and ovulation each cycle (although very occasionally more than one is released and fertilised, leading to non-identical twins or multiples!). This egg stays alive for twelve to twenty-four hours, and if it doesn't get fertilised by sperm, it disintegrates and is either reabsorbed by the body or shed with the lining of the uterus.

• **The hormone check-in** Both oestrogen and FSH levels have been increasing to this point, causing the ovarian follicles to develop, while oestrogen also prepares the uterus lining through growth and repair, helping to make it an ideal home for a fertilised egg. Hormonal changes cause cervical fluid to increase (offering the gift of natural lube and creating a friendlier environment for sperm). This cervical fluid is known as fertile discharge and is similar to egg whites; you can often start to notice it when you're looking out for it. And you may experience a slight rise in body temperature thanks to the LH surge. There's also a rise in testosterone (yep, it's not just guys who have this hormone), which is why you may feel increased sexual desire in the days before ovulation.

- **How fertile are you?** Spoiler alert: very. Ovulation is the 'main event' phase of the menstrual cycle. An egg is released from one ovary and travels down the fallopian tube. There are several DIY ways to assess whether you're ovulating, including tracking your cycle and assessing changes in your cervical mucus. Other methods include monitoring your temperature throughout your cycle using a specialist thermometer or using ovulation predictor sticks (at-home urine tests that detect the rise of the LH hormone which peaks just before ovulation). Some people notice other telltale signs during this phase, from feeling more energised, dynamic and motivated to less joyful physical symptoms like spotting, cramping or breast tenderness – all on account of your hormones.
- **How you might feel** With oestrogen rising you could feel more upbeat, optimistic and focused. You may also have an increased sex drive, which is an evolutionary way of encouraging sex for pregnancy (amazing, right?). Many women really enjoy this phase thanks to the increased oestrogen, and like to make the most of it. So, start your own company, run an ultramarathon or just tick off your to-do list and feel smug at getting your inbox to zero – if this is your time, lean into it.
- **Your to-do (or not-do) list** If you're interested in becoming pregnant, now and the few days leading up to ovulation

are your time to get it on (in official medical terms). If babies are not your vibe right now, continue to use your usual contraception or abstain from penetrative penis-in-vagina sex, and ride the feel-good hormone wave.

**A note on ovulating . . .**

Not every woman or person with a uterus ovulates, or ovulates every single cycle, during their reproductive years. Ovulation (and the menstrual cycle as a whole) can be made more unpredictable by age and stage of life, underlying medical conditions or illness, lifestyle factors, stress, medication or breastfeeding.

If you have a menstrual cycle without ovulating (this is called an 'anovulatory' cycle), pregnancy cannot occur, as an egg hasn't been released and therefore there is nothing for sperm to fertilise.

---

**Q:** I'm not on contraception, does getting my period (e.g. bleeding) mean that I've definitely ovulated?

We put this question to Dr Jerilynn C. Prior, Professor of Endocrinology and Metabolism at the University of British Columbia in Vancouver, Canada. She runs the UBC Centre for Menstrual Cycle and Ovulation Research (www.cemcor.ubc.ca). Jerilynn has spent her career studying menstrual cycles and the effects of the cycle's changing oestrogen and progesterone hormone levels on women's health. This was her response:

**A:** 'Although the assumption is that regular, normal-length menstrual cycles are always normally ovulatory, the reality is very different. To ovulate means to release an egg from the ovary and to make high levels of progesterone for at least ten and ideally twelve to fourteen days. Ovulatory disturbances, such as not ovulating (anovulation) and too short a duration of high progesterone (short luteal phase), are very common within normal-length cycles. Silent ovulatory disturbances (SOD) occur in a quarter to more than a third of all cycles according to a population-based study in Norway.[9] Cycles with ovulatory disturbances do not have normal fertility.

'Ovulation reflects women's well-being. That means that a woman who is belittled, abused, has the burden of a job at home and outside of the home, and lacks social emotional support is likely to develop SOD. If she is also not eating enough for her energy needs or becomes ill her cycles may also become longer than normal.[10] These adaptive changes are protective, since becoming pregnant when under those kinds of stressors is not good for the woman, her potential child or for her community. But that means that many of the "unexplained infertility" within regular cycles currently affecting almost 10 per cent of women could be prevented with a more supportive environment.'

---

### Phase 3: Luteal, after ovulation

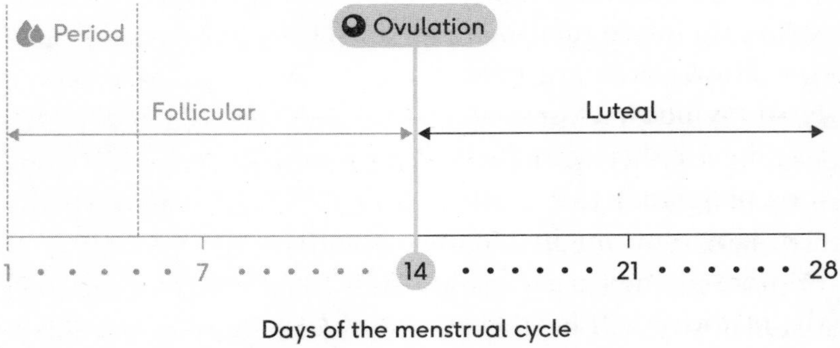


• **WTF is happening?** This marks roughly the second half of the cycle, the phase that begins the day after ovulation and continues until the day before your next period (unless fertilisation has taken place). During this time, the uterus readies itself to support the implantation of a fertilised egg and support a growing pregnancy.

• **The hormone check-in** After ovulation, the follicle that released the egg cleverly turns into a body of cells called the corpus luteum. The corpus luteum produces progesterone which maintains the perfect uterus lining for pregnancy by stimulating blood flow and glands that secrete nutrients. If the egg is not fertilised, and does not implant in the lining of the uterus, then the corpus luteum breaks down. Progesterone then falls, leading to contractions of the uterine muscles and the breakdown of its lining, which leaves the body as a period – and your cycle begins again. If fertilisation and implantation do occur, then progesterone continues to be released by the corpus luteum to maintain the uterus lining until the placenta takes over by the end of the first trimester. High progesterone levels need to remain throughout pregnancy to help support the developing pregnancy.

Importantly for how you feel, in this phase of the cycle, lower levels of oestrogen lead to a drop in other chemical messengers in the brain and body, such as dopamine and serotonin (often referred to as the happy hormones).

• **How fertile are you?** A day or so after ovulation, the fertile window closes. Typically, around a fortnight later, you'll get either your period or potentially a positive result on a pregnancy test.

• **How you might feel** Many of us will experience one or more premenstrual symptoms during this time but while the majority will be able to get on with day-to-day life, for others this is when premenstrual syndrome (PMS) or premenstrual dysphoric disorder (PMDD) can kick in. In which case you may feel filled with rage, exhaustion, depression or generally under the weather. Sad bonus points if all of the above describe this phase for you. The range of symptoms is vast, but common ones include cramps, fatigue, general aches and pains, bloating, breast tenderness, digestive issues with diarrhoea or constipation, zits and feeling irritable, anxious or low. No wonder it's sometimes described as 'period flu'. Needless to say, these less-than-sexy side effects mean that for many, sex drive is low during this time, and brain fog can make your usual everyday tasks a struggle.

• **Your to-do (or not-do) list** In Chapter 4, we look more closely at PMS and PMDD and how these are treated. If you're someone who suffers severely, it's worth speaking to your doctor about what might help. If you do experience this wave of unpleasant symptoms, try to make life as easy as possible for yourself during this time. If your appetite is up, having some healthy freezer meals ready can help free up brain space and time for things you want to do. This could be seeing your mates or embracing the joy of missing out for an early night, focusing on hobbies or exercise, having some outdoor time, or doing whatever you feel nurtures your brain best.

## Should you track your cycle?

There are useful medical reasons to track your menstrual cycle. It's a habit that can help you feel more 'in tune' with your body and recognise your usual pattern of symptoms or any irregularities. You can include any symptoms, like spotting or blood flow, cervical fluid, breast tenderness, etc., as well as other notables such as mood, pain and energy levels. Write it all down or record it in an app every day and within a few months you may notice a pattern – or if your hormones are more chaotic, at the very least you'll be able to observe this, and that's helpful to be aware of too.

It's also useful for many interactions you'll have with healthcare professionals, whether you want to use hormonal contraception, are trying to get a diagnosis for a medical condition like PCOS or endometriosis, or are trying to get pregnant.

### The origins of cycle tracking

Cycle tracking has become increasingly digitised in recent years, with a rise in apps collecting your period and cycle data. Before then, the trusty pen and paper calendar helped many of us keep tabs. And before that? Millennia ago, it seems we may have had some pretty inventive ways of monitoring fertility. Take the Ishango Bone – this mammal fibula (possibly a baboon's) was found in 1950 during the years of Belgian colonial rule in the Democratic Republic of Congo before it became independent. The Ishango Bone is thought to be more than 20,000 years old. What makes it fascinating is the small notch markings carved into it, showing a very early form of mathematics. This is widely regarded to be a primitive type of calendar and some speculate it was a woman's doing, as a way to track her cycle. Though there isn't a way to prove this, we can well believe this was the work of an early period-tracking pioneer.

## How do synthetic hormones in contraception affect your cycle?

You've had a glimpse into the hormonal rollercoaster that naturally supports your menstrual cycle. But when it comes to hormonal contraception, you might be wondering how hormones which naturally prepare the body for pregnancy can also be used in contraception to *prevent* it.

Every type of hormonal contraception contains a synthetic version of the hormone progesterone, which is called progestin. We tend to use the word 'progestogen' as a catch-all term, which refers to both natural progesterone and synthetic progestin. Progestin was originally created by scientists in the 1950s with a view to treating gynaecological conditions, and then went on to be used in contraception. The need for progestin came about when scientists discovered that natural progesterone, when taken orally, is ineffective as it is processed by the liver (and removed as waste rather than acting where you want it to).[11] This meant a suitable alternative had to be found. Different types of progestin affect the body in widely different ways, and because their side effects are so varied from person to person, there have been many generations developed in the decades that have followed the first iterations – all in the hope of designing a more beneficial synthetic form of progesterone.

Progestin and oestrogen used in contraception have a 'negative feedback effect' on the hormonal changes in the menstrual cycle. Negative feedback is when high levels of a hormone block the release of another hormone. Taking synthetic oestrogen and progestin in hormonal contraception causes negative feedback by blocking the release of the hormones that control the menstrual cycle (LH and FSH) from the pituitary gland. This means you may not have menstrual cycles while using some types of hormonal contraception (the low dose of progestin in hormonal coils and some progestogen-only pills are exceptions to this, see Chapter 5). Hormonal contraceptives may work to:

- Prevent ovulation, stopping the cascade of hormonal changes required to develop follicles and release a mature egg.
- Affect the production of cervical fluid, ensuring it's not 'fertile quality' and that it's too thick for sperm to pass through, preventing sperm from entering the uterus. This is similar to the type of cervical mucus during the progesterone-dominant luteal phase.
- Ensure the lining of the uterus remains too thin for a fertilised egg to implant into by preventing the usual build-up of blood vessels and tissue during the phases of the menstrual cycle.[12]

Synthetic oestrogen and progestin can interact with other hormones and our natural biological system in loads of different ways, meaning side effects can be hard to predict and wide ranging. Some women may be sensitive to synthetic oestrogen, but it's often the progestin that's the issue. Your stage of life can also play a huge part in how you react to progestin, as it behaves differently while interacting with your ever-changing hormonal profile throughout your reproductive life, such as after pregnancy, in perimenopause or after menopause. As you might expect, past research is limited and given many of the studies looking into progestin were carried out on small mammals (with results then extrapolated to humans), they're not particularly helpful.

In Chapters 2 and 3, we look more closely at hormonal contraception.

# 2

# The pill

It doesn't matter if you're sixteen, twenty-six or beyond, this chapter is for anyone considering going on the pill for the first time, those in need of a refresher, or if you want to learn how the pill actually works. You may also be wondering about the difference between the main types of pills, and why there are so many different names anyway? Let's get into it.

If you're new to hormonal contraception, the method that you've probably already heard about is the pill. Often, we hear women say, 'When I was sixteen, I was *put on* the pill', not, 'I *chose* to go on the pill.' This language suggests some autonomy is taken away from us when it comes to going on the pill for the first time – a stark difference from the liberating rhetoric of the 1960s when it was first introduced. Many of us might feel this way now because our feelings have changed towards the pill due to experiencing unwanted side effects, or we just didn't know what other contraceptives were out there, so how did we know how to ask about them? There's a reason the pill is so commonly prescribed when you first decide to use hormonal contraception. It's cheap to prescribe, accessible, highly effective, and it's easy to start and stop. For context, older pills like Microgynon and Levest cost the NHS less than £3 every three months. While newer pills, like Yasmin and Lucette, can cost almost £15 (which is still far cheaper than raising a child!).

So for a long time, generations (Gen X and Millennials, in particular) have been prescribed the pill; some taking it for years – even decades – without necessarily engaging with what's in it and how it affects their bodies or mood. While the pill has done amazing things for body autonomy and women's liberation, many of us may well hold preconceptions about it. This is usually based on years of misinformation that has let down generations of pill users, or would-be users; and we've seen a rise in misinformation due to social media. So throughout this chapter, we'll be swapping the lore for science as we include some of the most common queries our Lowdown doctors are asked.

First, we'll delve into how the pill works to prevent pregnancy, along with the types and brands available. We'll help you get your head around your options – because there's more than you might think – and the best way to use it effectively. So hopefully, when you're done reading you'll know more about your pill than the colour of its packaging (not a dig, we see this a lot).

## What even *is* the pill?

Is there any other medication that goes by such a generic term, yet is immediately recognisable?

Oral contraceptives (aka the pill) are taken by around 150 million people around the world, for contraception and/or to manage health conditions.[1] Developed in the 1950s and released in (some) countries in 1960, it became available to married women only in the UK on the NHS in 1961. It's difficult to underestimate the significance of the pill, not only in terms of its medical benefits but also the major social change it brought with it. A bastion of female empowerment, it didn't just allow for sex with fewer consequences, but it led to more women finishing education and entering the workforce. It wasn't plain sailing, though; there were cultural or religious objections – in some countries it was deemed the end of civilised society, leading to immorality and the decline of a woman's place in the home, meaning it was banned. However you look at it, it had a transformative effect on our reproductive health, family planning – and the ability to control both. Over sixty years later, it is the most commonly used form of hormonal contraception, which in much of the world is accessible, cost-effective and with high rates of effectiveness.

In the decades that have followed its release, there have been many, many versions of the original pill, containing different types of hormones in varying levels. And yet, fundamentally, it really hasn't changed much. This lack of development hasn't been serving us well, particularly those who want an effective contraceptive but may struggle with side effects. In Chapter 12, we look at the future of hormonal contraception and whether radical change is on the horizon.

### A controversial history

Though we have benefited hugely from the early innovation in contraceptive development, it's important to acknowledge that the history of contraception is deeply entwined with the history of racism and eugenics (the concept that selective breeding improves the genetic quality of the human race).

Margaret Sanger was an early advocate of bringing contraception to the masses and popularised the term 'birth control'. She opened America's first contraceptive clinic in 1916 and founded Planned Parenthood, a non-profit that continues to provide sexual healthcare to millions. However, she was also a believer in eugenics. The author Angela Davis explains in her book *Women, Race and Class* that Sanger used birth control as a way to control the population of those she deemed 'unfit', including people of colour, immigrants and poor communities. (Note that the Planned Parenthood organisation has disavowed Sanger, citing her past record with eugenics and racism.)

Co-inventor of the combined oral contraceptive pill, Gregory Pincus, used Puerto Rico as a testing ground for his large-scale human trial of the pill.[2] There were many ethical and safety contraventions with the trial, not least the fact that the Puerto Rican women who took part in the study were only told they were taking a drug that prevented pregnancy, not that it was a clinical trial with potential risks. The pill, called Enovid, contained high doses of hormones, which led to numerous side effects reported by 17 per cent of the women.[3] Pincus ignored these, dismissing many as 'psychosomatic'. Twenty-five women dropped out of the study due to side effects and, shockingly, three women died during the trials.

This dark history casts a shadow over the contraceptive advancements of the twentieth century. As we move forward, reproductive justice advocates campaign to ensure all women have access to safe and effective contraception without coercion or discrimination.

## So, how does it work?

The pill contains synthetic hormones which mimic the natural hormones in your body. You can read more in Chapter

1 about how the hormones in the pill affect your menstrual cycle and work to prevent pregnancy by stopping ovulation, thickening cervical mucus and thinning the uterus lining.

Taken perfectly, it is very effective at preventing pregnancy, and for many who take it to ease period problems and symptoms of other conditions, it has a life-changing impact on their everyday well-being. On the other hand, taking a pill everyday doesn't work for everyone. And for those taking a pill, or another type of hormonal contraception that doesn't agree with them, the negative side effects can be frustrating – which is why finding one that works better for you can be crucial.

## Is the pill really 99 per cent effective? Typical vs. perfect use explained

When taken correctly the pill is over 99 per cent effective. But what does this actually mean and does this stat reflect real life and the potential for human error? When we talk about contraception effectiveness, you'll often come across the terms 'typical use' versus 'perfect use'. 'Perfect use' is what we see in clinical trials, where researchers have prompted and ensured that participants take the method correctly all the time. This can give a false assurance of how effective a method is, because it doesn't take into account the hot mess that is human nature, meaning it's unlikely most of us will use a method perfectly all the time. For instance, if you're unable to take your pill at your usual time because travel plans have messed up your schedule, or you miss it altogether because you didn't bring it on a weekend away, this can impact its effectiveness. Which brings us to 'typical use'. Typical use is what we think of as real-world use, and for that reason, it's the one we tend to care most about. This includes all the pregnancies which happen when people were using contraception regardless of how reliably they were using it. So, in reality, typical use effectiveness for the pill is actually more like 91–93 per cent, meaning around 7–9 in 100 users will get pregnant each year.[4]

## What can make the pill less effective?

• **Vomiting and diarrhoea** Whether you're ill or feeling rough after a big night, vomiting can interfere with the pill's effectiveness. If you do vomit within three hours of taking your pill, follow the missed pill rules on 51–54. Similarly, the pill's effectiveness can be reduced by diarrhoea that's been ongoing for twenty-four hours or more.

• **Medication** If you need to take any other medications while on the pill, always check with your healthcare professional that they're compatible with the hormonal contraception you're using. Some medications can increase the speed that the pill is used up in your body, so can make it less effective. These medications include unusual antibiotics (used to treat conditions such as tuberculosis), some anti-epilepsy medications and some migraine medications. This applies to herbal or homeopathic remedies too, such as St John's wort. So please tell your doctor, nurse or pharmacist if you use any medications or supplements so they can check for interactions. It may be necessary to switch to another method or use additional protection, such as condoms, if you are using a medication that prevents the pill from working properly. The combined pill can, in turn, affect other medications – important ones being thyroxine used to treat thyroid problems and epilepsy medications like lamotrigine. Lamotrigine can reduce the effectiveness of some contraceptives and, in turn, contraceptives may alter how lamotrigine works, so please start, stop and switch methods under the guidance of a healthcare professional. The pill can potentially increase the amount of thyroxine you need to take, so it's a good idea to have your thyroid levels checked six weeks after starting the pill if you take thyroxine.[5]

## What are the main types of pill?

If you've already done even a small amount of research into choosing a contraceptive pill, you may have seen dozens of different options. It can feel overwhelming at first, but let's scale it back a bit. There are two main categories of contraceptive pill available, the first contains a combination of synthetic oestrogen and progestin, and the other is just progestin.

### Combined pill

Over 99 per cent effective with perfect use; around 91–93 per cent effective with typical use.[6]

Overall satisfaction rating: ★★★☆☆ **2.8**/5 from 2,468 reviews

As rated by users at thelowdown.com

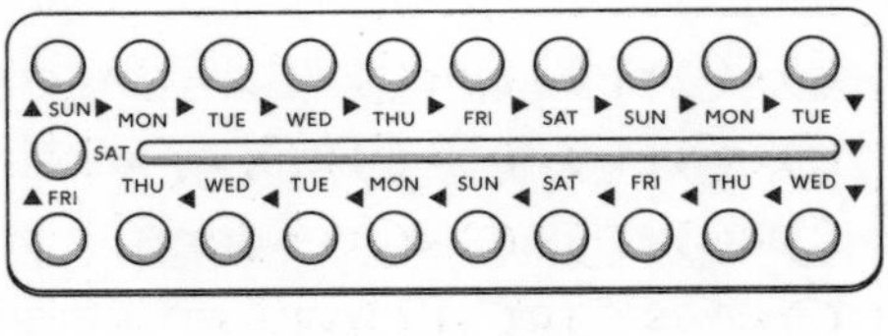


**Combined pill**

This contains synthetic versions of both oestrogen and progesterone. The combined pill is often the type of contraceptive pill that you are first prescribed. It's a daily pill that you should take at roughly the same time each day. There are different types of oestrogen and progestogen and varying concentrations of each of these hormones in the numerous combined pill brands available. Pills can be 'monophasic', meaning they contain the same hormone concentration in every pill in the packet, or 'multiphasic', where the concentrations of hormones can vary throughout the packet. Traditionally, users were advised to take a packet of the combined pill followed by a planned break from the hormones of up to seven days, during which you would expect to have a bleed. However, in modern times, you can use the combined pill in different ways, referred to as 'tailored use', which we'll talk about shortly. Some packets have placebo, sugar or reminder pills as a built in break, these may be called ED or 'every day' pills.

## Progestogen-only pill (aka POP or mini pill)

Over 99 per cent effective with perfect use; around 91–93 per cent effective with typical use.[7]

Overall satisfaction rating: ★ ★ ★ ☆ ☆ 2.7/5 from 1,301 reviews

As rated by users at thelowdown.com

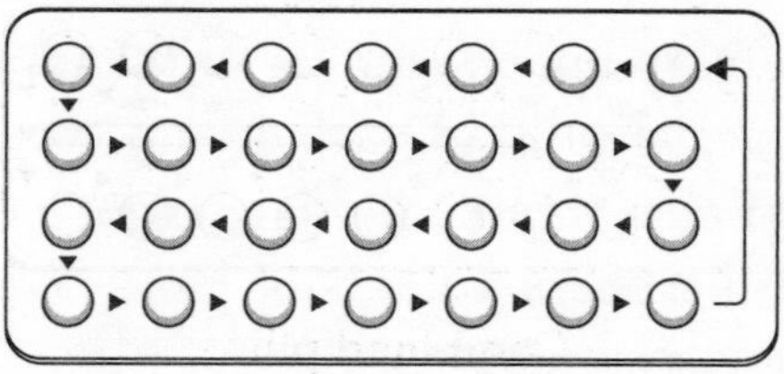

**Progestogen-only pill**

The clue is in the name here; this type of contraceptive pill contains progestogen without any oestrogen. It's often used by people who are unable to use combined contraception that contains oestrogen, which isn't medically safe for everyone. You must take it every day within three, twelve, or twenty-four hours of your usual time (depending on the type of progestogen-only pill) for it to still be effective.

## What are the different pill brands?

Now you've got the basics down, let's go a little further.

The main pill types – combined and progestogen-only – can be then further categorised into pill groups, depending on their ingredients, i.e. which synthetic hormones they contain.

With dozens of pill brands on the market, and many brand names containing the exact same hormonal ingredients but packaged differently, it's no wonder people get confused. There are seventeen groups of combined pills and four groups of progestogen-only pill currently on the market in the UK, but because there are multiple brand names within each of these groups, the majority of people think that each pill is different. However, they're often the same generic pill but with new names. For example, Microgynon, Ovranette, Rigevidon and Levest (brand names) contain the same synthetic hormones: ethinylestradiol (a type of oestrogen) and levonorgestrel (a type of progestogen) in the same doses.

Once you gain an understanding of the type and strength of hormones in the pills in each group, you can research the brands available where you live. Now let's get into the specifics. Warning: there are lots of long medical names for different hormones coming up.

### The Lowdown on the combined pill groups

There are two main things that vary between types of combined pill:

- The **oestrogen:** most combined pills contain synthetic oestrogen called ethinylestradiol in varying strengths. In recent years, four new brands of pill have been developed that each contain a new type of oestrogen.
- The **progestogen:** there are many different types of progestogen used in pills which may have slightly different side effects and are often described as being more or less 'androgenic' or 'anti-androgenic' (explained below).

Overleaf is a table that summarises the main groups of combined pill available in the UK and Ireland at the time of writing. Traditionally, every pill used the same type of synthetic oestrogen (ethinylestradiol) in varying concentrations. Low-oestrogen pills contain 20 micrograms of ethinylestradiol, standard or medium-oestrogen pills contain 30 micrograms, and high-oestrogen pills contain 35 micrograms. Your healthcare professional can change your pill brand based on the side effects you may be experiencing. For example, if you're experiencing heavy bleeding or lots of breakthrough bleeding (unscheduled bleeding when you're not expecting it) on one pill, then switching to a pill with a higher concentration of ethinylestradiol may help to control it. However, if you experience symptoms like bloating, breast pain, nausea, headaches or low libido, which can be side effects caused by oestrogen, you could try switching to a lower oestrogen pill to see if these improve. The pills Norinyl-1, Qlaira, Zoely and Drovelis, contain different types of oestrogen which are more similar to that naturally produced by your body, but there is not enough evidence (yet) to suggest this makes much difference in terms of side effects.

If you experience side effects that are more related to the progestogen within the pill brand – such as acne, anxiety, low mood or vaginal dryness – you can try a different brand containing a more or less androgenic progestogen.

## Combined pill groups

| Group | Oestrogen type | Oestrogen level | Progestogen type |
|---|---|---|---|
| 1 | Ethinylestradiol | Low | Levonorgestrel |
| 2 | | Low | Desogestrel |
| 3 | | Low | Gestodene |
| 4 | | Low | Drospirenone |
| 5 | | Medium | Levonorgestrel |
| 6 | | Medium | Desogestrel |
| 7 | | Medium | Gestodene |
| 8 | | Medium | Drospirenone |
| 9 | | High | Norethisterone (1mg) |
| 10 | | High | Norethisterone (0.5mg) |
| 11 | | High | Levonorgestrel |
| 12 | | High | Norgestimate |
| 13 | | High | Co-cyprindiol |
| 14 | Mestranol | Can't compare | Norethisterone |
| 15 | Estradiol valerate | Can't compare | Dienogest |
| 16 | Estradiol hemihydrate | Can't compare | Nomegestrol |
| 17 | Estetrol monohydrate | Can't compare | Drospirenone |

| **Progestogen androgenicity** | **Combined pill brand names** |
|---|---|
| Androgenic | Leonore, Microlite |
| Less androgenic | Bimizza, Gedarel 20/150, Mercilon |
| Less androgenic | Akizza 20/75, Femodette, Millinette 20/75, Sunya |
| Anti-androgenic | Eloine, Yasminelle, Yaz |
| Androgenic | Ambelina, Elevin, Levest, Maexini, Microgynon, Microgynon ED, Ovranette, Ovreena, Rigevidon |
| Less androgenic | Cimizt, Gedarel 30/150, Marvelon, Marviol, Minulet |
| Less androgenic | Akizza 30/75, Femodene, Femodene ED, Katya, Millinette 30/75 |
| Anti-androgenic | Dretine, Lucette, Yacella, Yasmin |
| Androgenic | Norimin, Synphase |
| Androgenic | Brevinor |
| Androgenic | Logynon, Logynon ED, TriRegol |
| Less androgenic | Lizinna |
| Anti-androgenic | Clairette, Dianette |
| Androgenic | Norinyl-1 |
| Anti-androgenic | Qlaira |
| Anti-androgenic | Zoely |
| Anti-androgenic | Drovelis |

The Lowdown website 2024

**Combined pill review**
Used for 6-12 months 18 years old

★★★★☆

**Brevinor pill**

My favourite combined pill so far! My periods used to be super-heavy and around eleven days long, I'd vomit . . . etc. I have tried Rigevidon and Yasmin but found that they affected my moods quite negatively. This one has higher oestrogen. My periods now last four days and I only get light cramps for a day! I go through the normal cycles of my boobs hurting the week before my period, which I never had before. My mood feels a lot more stable on this pill too. My skin has always been clear and this pill hasn't changed that. I do find that I have more headaches but I'm not sure if I'm just taking notice more.

Shared on **thelowdown.com**

## What are androgens?

Androgens are a group of sex hormones, which includes testosterone. They're commonly associated with men but are also found in women's bodies too, just in lower concentrations. High levels of androgens in women may cause acne, excessive body hair and balding. These can also be symptoms of a condition called polycystic ovary syndrome (PCOS), which is associated with high levels of androgens.

All hormonal contraception contains synthetic progestogen. Because synthetic progestogens are similar to testosterone, some can bind with androgen receptors in our cells and either block or activate them. A progestogen is considered androgenic if it triggers an androgenic response in the body, which leads to the types of side effects mentioned above. Natural progesterone (the kind that our bodies make) is actually anti-androgenic, and the most recent generations of synthetic progestogens have been developed in an attempt to create progestogens that do not have an androgenic effect. Progestogens can be described as 'androgenic' or 'anti-androgenic' – but the reality is that they often fall somewhere between the two extremes.

Androgenic strength

| Progestogen | Androgenic strength |
| --- | --- |
| Levonorgestrel | Most androgenic |
| Norethisterone<br>Norethisterone Enanthate<br>Norelgestromin | Androgenic |
| Nomegestrol Acetate | Mildly androgenic |
| Norgestimate<br>Medroxyprogesterone Acetate<br>Gestodene<br>Etonogestrel<br>Desogestrel | Less androgenic |
| Drospirenone<br>Natural progesterone | Anti-androgenic |

Understanding the androgenic effects of your contraception is complex. So, if you have concerns about the impact of your method, or any of the side effects, speak to your GP.

## Progestogen-only pill groups

Like the combined pill, there are many brands of progestogen-only pill out there. Not all progestogen-only pills are the same, as you may have guessed by now. These groups are much simpler than the combined pill groups, as there are only four different groups of progestogen-only pill in the UK.

### Progestogen-only pill groups

| Group | Progestogen type | Progestogen androgenicity | Brand names |
|---|---|---|---|
| 1 | Desogestrel | Less androgenic | Aizea, Cerazette, Cerelle, Desogestrel, Desomono, Desorex, Feonolla, Hana, Lovima, Zelleta |
| 2 | Norethisterone | Androgenic | Noriday |
| 3 | Levonorgestrel | Androgenic | Norgeston |
| 4 | Drospirenone | Anti-androgenic | Slynd |

The Lowdown website 2024

- **Desogestrel** is the synthetic progestin used in the most common progestogen-only pill.
- **Traditional** progestogen-only pills are older pills containing levonorgestrel or norethisterone.
- **Drospirenone** is the synthetic progestin used in a newer type of progestogen-only pill under the brand name Slynd.

Traditional progestogen-only pills work predominantly by changing the cervical mucus to make it harder for sperm to get through, and by thinning the uterus lining so a fertilised egg can't implant. They don't reliably stop ovulation for everyone so some women may still have a menstrual cycle while taking these pills, but this doesn't impact the contraceptive effect. In general, the newer types of pill tend to be preferred over the traditional types, because they do stop ovulation, and give you a longer window in which to remember to take them, offering more leeway than the traditional progestogen-only pills. (See 'Do I need to take the pill at the same time each day' below.)

---

**Q:** I don't like the idea of taking something unnatural long term – or am I overthinking it?

**A:** You can safely take the combined pill until you're fifty, and the progestogen-only pill until fifty-five when contraception is no longer needed, if you're otherwise well. And for most people the benefits will outweigh the risks[8] (more on this in Chapter 6). But how long you want to stay on the pill is a completely individual choice. There are pros and cons of taking the pill, and it's all about the balance for you. If the pill is still beneficial for you, then of course you can keep taking it, however, if your circumstances or side effects change you have plenty of other options.

---

## Which pill should I choose?

While no one expects you to be an expert on every single pill brand, it's helpful to know your options, especially if you're looking to manage other symptoms, like acne, as well as choosing a contraceptive. Having an overview of the ingredients in each pill group can help you prepare for your appointment. Whether you take the combined pill or progestogen-only pill. it's often found that different pills work better for different people, so there may be some trial and error involved.

Anecdotally we sometimes find people experience a change in side effects when switching between pill brands which contain exactly the same hormonal ingredients at exactly the same doses, for example from Cerazette to Hana or vice versa. We don't know exactly why this happens as there is no research into this, but it may be due to the other non-active/non-hormonal ingredients contained within the pills, called the 'excipients'. If you've experienced this, please know that you're not the only one!

**Progestogen only/mini pill**
Used for 6–12 months 33 years old

★☆☆☆☆

**Cerelle pill**

After being on another mini pill for years without issue (Cerazette) I was put on Cerelle unexpectedly. Immediately I started feeling nauseous and dizzy, fatigued and generally incredibly low to the point where I had to take time off work. My mood didn't improve for the nine months I was on this pill and I lost all interest in sex, experienced vaginal dryness, and all I wanted to do was sleep. The symptoms were so bad my doctor thought I had a thyroid issue, but tests all came back normal. As soon as I stopped taking Cerelle the symptoms dramatically improved.

Shared on **thelowdown.com**

**Q:** I've recently started taking the combined pill and my boobs have become sore and tender. What's going on?!

**A:** The struggle is real. On The Lowdown, tender or enlarged breasts are the most commonly reported side effect of all hormonal contraceptives. It's pretty common to experience an increase in boob size when you start hormonal contraception as oestrogen and/or progestogen can cause fluid retention. Your boobs should go back to normal within a few months of starting your method (or if you decide to stop using it). If your boobs are feeling sore, over-the-counter painkillers such as paracetamol or ibuprofen or supplements containing an essential fatty acid called gamma linolenic acid like starflower oil or evening primrose oil may help. If your boobs remain sore and tender you could try switching to a lower oestrogen pill, progestogen-only method or non-hormonal option. Breast pain is not a typical symptom of breast cancer but if you notice other changes like any new lumps or bumps, or changes in skin texture or colour, always get it checked out by a healthcare professional.

---

## Where to get the pill

In the UK hormonal contraceptives are available on prescription for free on the NHS via GP surgeries, contraception or sexual health clinics, and some young people's services. At the time of writing, the NHS is rolling out access to oral contraceptive pills in community pharmacies in England, which means these will be free from your pharmacist and just require a short consultation. Thanks to these changes, you can also now order your contraception for free on the NHS via The Lowdown's online service. There are also two types of progestogen-only pills (Hana and Lovima) that do not require prescriptions and can be bought in pharmacies over the counter. You also have the option of buying your contraception through a private clinic or online pharmacy.

## How will I feel when starting the pill?

When it's your first time taking the pill, there may be an element of suck-it-and-see, as we all respond differently to the types and levels of hormones used in the pill. While some won't feel much, if any, difference taking the pill than not taking it, others will have side effects ranging from mild to severe. In one survey conducted by Channel 4 with over 4,000 responses, almost 80 per cent of users experienced side effects from hormonal contraceptives.[9] However, it is important to recognise that there could be some bias in this statistic as women who are having side effects may be more likely to respond to these surveys. Nevertheless, when women say they are having side effects from hormonal contraceptives, at The Lowdown, we listen. We'll look more closely at some of the most common side effects in Chapter 5, which can include things like changes to mood, libido and vaginal discharge and dryness, not to mention period-like cramps and lower back pain, nausea, skin breakouts, breast tenderness and enlargement (the list goes on).

But there are some lesser-known side effects too, reported to us by Lowdown users, and some are pretty weird. Take contact lens sensitivity, for example. Oral contraception can reduce the amount of tears you produce, making contacts less comfortable.[10] If you're sensitive to the different progestogens within certain hormonal contraceptives, it can trigger hair loss and a small minority of users may experience some of their hair falling out.

When starting your first pill or switching to a new type, keep tabs on any changes you feel in your body or your mood. Keeping a list of these, and how they might ebb and flow day to day, will help you tune into the effects your pill is having and whether it's the right fit for you. If you're going on the pill to help with cycle-related issues like mood swings or heavy periods, take a note of your symptoms before starting the pill (rating them out of 10 for severity); this will give you a really easy way to compare if they've improved once you start taking the pill. Healthcare professionals usually recommend waiting for three months in case side effects ease, after which if you do need to switch it up, you will have a ready-to-go record of your symptoms to discuss with your GP.

## How do I start the pill?

Most people can begin taking the pill at any time during their cycle. If you start taking most combined or progestogen-only pills on days one to five of your period you will be protected from pregnancy straight away.[11] If you start the pill after day five of your period (or after day one for some combined pills), you will be advised to avoid sex or use condoms for the first seven days of taking the combined pill or drospirenone progestogen-only pill, or two days if starting the desogestrel or a traditional progestogen-only pill. In most cases you can start contraception straight away after having a baby, miscarriage or an abortion, and you'll be protected against pregnancy immediately. If you start contraception more than twenty-one days after giving birth or more than five days after a miscarriage or abortion you'll need to use extra protection as described above.

---

**Q:** If I'm taking the pill, do I still have a 'normal' menstrual cycle and do I ovulate?

**A:** The combined pill and the newer versions of the progestogen-only pill stop you from ovulating. Therefore, you don't have a menstrual cycle. In fact, the bleed that you experience when you have a break from the combined pill is *not* a period; it's called a withdrawal bleed and is caused by the sudden drop of synthetic hormones in your bloodstream. This is why we say that periods on the combined pill are not 'real' periods, as they aren't caused by the same natural hormone changes. Withdrawal bleeding cannot be used as a reliable indicator that you're not pregnant. If you've missed pills or suspect you could be pregnant, take a pregnancy test. During these scheduled breaks from the hormones in the pill you may also experience some side effects that can be similar to PMS symptoms, but again, these are caused by the drop in levels of hormones when you stop taking the pill every day. The exception is for traditional progestogen-only pills where some women may still ovulate so may still have cyclical symptoms.

---

## Do you need to take the pill at the same time each day?

It's best to take your pill at the same time every day, or as close as possible. If this time no longer works for you, it's possible to change the time you take your pill so long as you adhere to the 'safe window' for the type you're taking.

Everyone is advised to take their pill around the same time each day to maintain its effectiveness and prevent side effects like breakthrough or irregular bleeding. If you deviate from your usual time (but it's still within the safe window for that pill type), it is classed as a 'late pill'. As long as you take your pill within the safe window, you'll still be protected against pregnancy – it's this safe window that also allows you to tweak the timings of your pill.

On the other hand, a 'missed pill' is where the timeframe in which you haven't taken your pill exceeds the safe window. This means you may not be protected from pregnancy. There's more info on how to work out whether you need to take emergency contraception in Chapter 8.

Your safe window will vary depending on the type of pill you're taking. Here are the headlines:

- **Combined pill** The safe window for this type of pill is twenty-four hours, i.e. you need to take your pill within twenty-four hours of the time that you should have taken it (or within forty-eight hours of taking your last pill). A pill is considered 'missed' once you exceed a window of twenty-four hours or more beyond when you should have taken your pill (see overleaf for a helpful illustrative example). This is longer than most progestogen-only pills so, you have more leeway with the combined pill, meaning it can be a good option if your schedule is less flexible.

Safe window

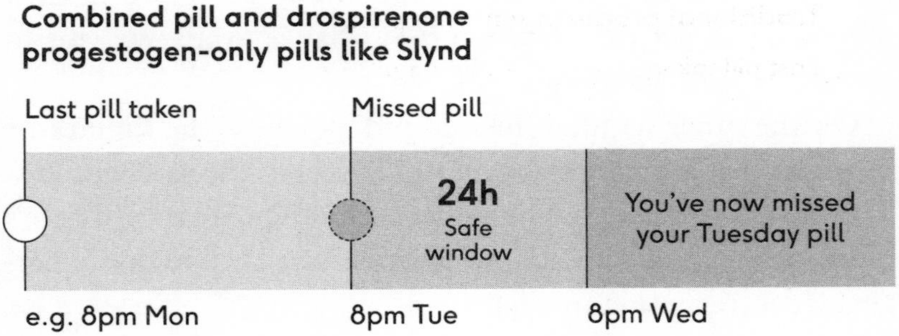


• **Progestogen-only pill** Missing just one progestogen-only pill can reduce the effectiveness and may mean you can become pregnant if you've had unprotected sex. Depending on the type of progestogen-only pill, the safe window is either three (traditional progestogen-only pills), twelve (desogestrel progestogen-only pills) or twenty-four (drospirenone progestogen-only pills) hours. The best way to change progestogen-only pills with a three-hour window is to gradually adapt to a new time in two- or three-hour blocks (e.g. Monday 10 a.m., Tuesday noon, Wednesday 2 p.m., and so on). If you need to switch sooner, just use another contraceptive (like a condom) as a back-up until you've been taking the pill for a full two days at your new time.

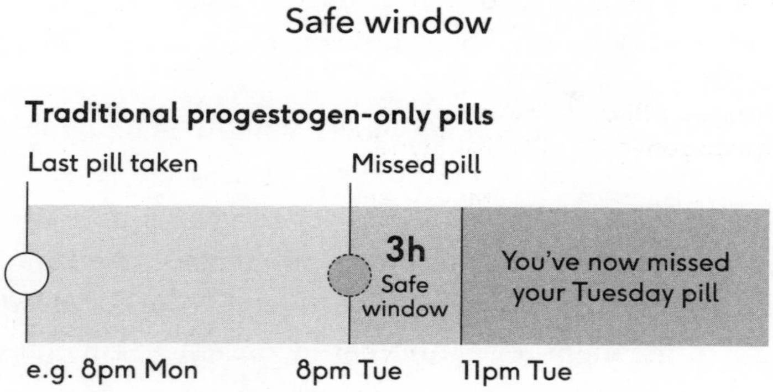


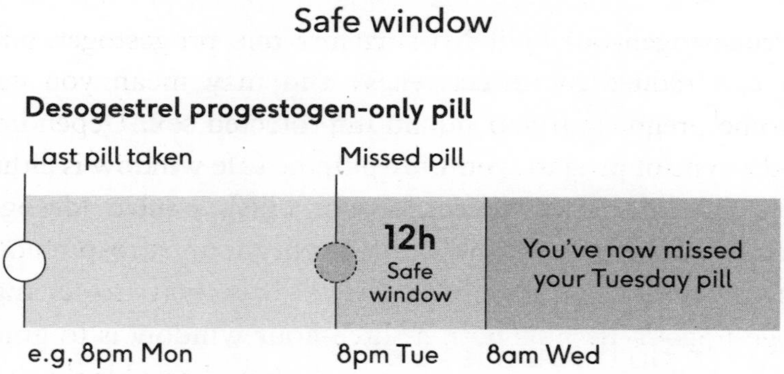


If you do struggle to remember to take the pill when you should, consider trying out 'habit stacking'. Productivity gurus often recommend habit stacking for when you are trying to ingrain a habit into your day-to-day life, so that it becomes second nature and you no longer have to think about it. It involves piggybacking your new habit onto an existing one. So, you might always take your pill before you brush your teeth in the morning, or just after you wash your face at night. In the next chapter, we look at other methods of hormonal contraception, which are longer lasting and don't require daily action like pill-taking. These are often popular because they're not an added chore to tick off the daily to-do list. So if you're constantly snoozing your pill alarm or scrambling to take it on time, don't worry, there are other options out there for you that contain the same ingredients as many pills.

If you're off on a holiday where you'll be changing time zones, remembering to take the pill at the right time can be confusing. The easiest way is to try to keep a note of your usual time so that you take your pill at the same time you would at home. If this means you'd have to wake up in the middle of the night, or at another inconvenient time, follow the advice on safe windows. For the super-organised, you might even consider gradually adapting your pill time in the weeks before your holiday in order to make it more convenient to take while you're away. You can also double up with another method, like condoms, to tide you over.

There's no need to worry when the clocks go forwards and back, as a one-hour difference won't affect when you need to take your pill.

## What to do if you miss a pill

If you've missed a pill using the safe window definitions above, we know it can be pretty tricky to interpret the humongous patient information leaflet to work out what to do. So rather than rewriting that prose within this book, we suggest you go straight to our handy online tool. We used the latest guidance from the Faculty of Sexual and Reproductive Healthcare (FSRH) and the pill manufacturers to create an online algorithm, taking the stress out of an already stressful situation. So please head over to the thelowdown.com/missed-pill for easy to understand instructions. You'll also find a handy QR code in the Resources section.

## Can you take the pill continuously without a break?

If you take a progestogen-only pill (apart from drospirenone-based pill Slynd) you'll never take a break, so just keep popping those pills. The combined pill, however, usually follows a '21/7 format', so twenty-one days on the pill, seven days break, then repeat. As previously mentioned, some pills say 'ED' after the name, meaning 'every day' – these contain a number of 'dummy' sugar (called placebo or reminder) pills, which mimic the seven-day break – you keep taking a tablet every day and will usually have a scheduled bleed during this time. Other combined pills and the progestogen-only pill Slynd come in pill packets with twenty-eight pills including dummy pills to build in a shorter break of two to four days during which you normally have a bleed. You can actually take the combined pill continuously without the break in order to skip a bleed. We explain more about how to do this and how to use contraception to skip your period, in Chapter 4.

**Combined pill**
Used for 6-12 months · 20 years old

★★★★★

**Rigevidon**

I was weary to go on Rigevidon after switching from a mini pill that caused non-stop bleeding and decreased sex drive, however, I was positively surprised. For me, I found the side effects minimal if not positive: clearer skin and slightly bigger boobs. I take it without a break, which means I only bleed every few months and find it a convenient method of contraception.

Shared on **thelowdown.com**

---

**Q:** Given there are lots of different types of hormonal contraception out there, why will my GP most likely default to prescribing the pill? Can I ask for a different method?

**A:** Of course you can ask for a different method, and a healthcare professional should discuss all available methods with you. GPs shouldn't default to the pill, but the pill is often the one that first-time contraceptive users default to themselves. Why? This is perhaps a generational thing, as our parents may have only known about or used the pill, so as we discuss contraception with them, they immediately lean more towards the pill. It can also be due to the additional benefits of the pill, including treatment for heavy or irregular periods and acne, which usually affect teenagers who are also looking to choose a contraceptive for the first time. Pills are also easier to start and stop than other methods. As contraceptive pills become more widely available on the NHS in community pharmacies we might find that easier access through high-street and online pharmacies, rather than waiting for a GP or a sexual health clinic appointment, means pills will be an even more popular choice.

# 3

# Alternatives to the pill

We've looked at the power of the pill as the predominant form of hormonal contraception around the world. While it's the undisputed trailblazer of hormonal contraception, many are surprised when they hear there are other contraceptive options out there.

The timeline opposite shows the various methods of hormonal and non-hormonal contraception and roughly when they were made available in the UK. At first glance it seems as though we've had lots of innovation. But the combined pill, ring and patch are pretty much exactly the same thing, containing the same types of hormones; they're just administered into our bodies differently. The same goes with the progestogen-only pill, implant, hormonal coil and injection. The scientific mode of action behind these methods is the same. These methods do, however, contain varying types and amounts of progestogen, which can behave in conflicting ways in the body and have the potential to make women feel very different while using each method. Natural Cycles, the first app cleared for use as a digital contraceptive, has actually been one of the biggest developments we've had in the last twenty years. And this is closely modelled on an existing non-hormonal method of natural family planning, called the symptothermal method.

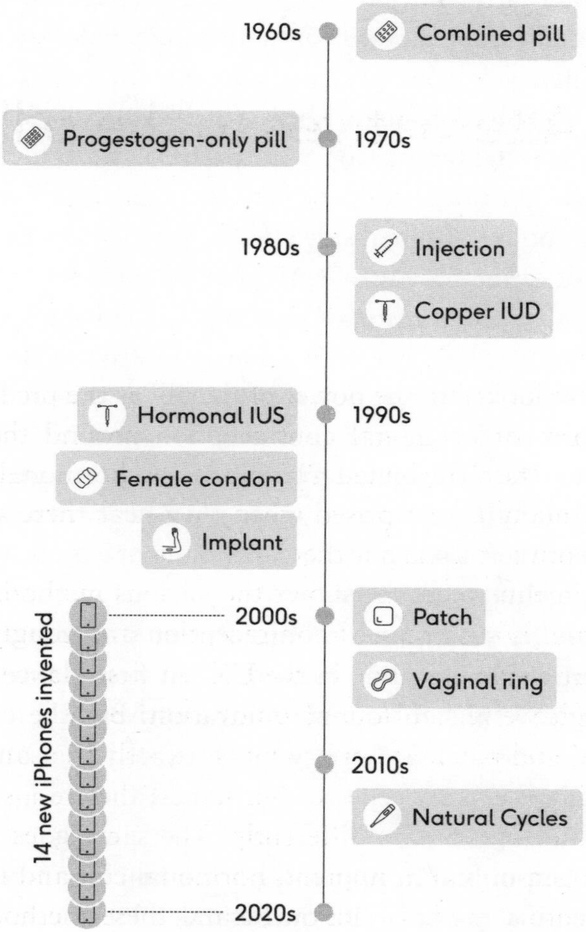


A huge lack of investment means there have been more versions of the iPhone created in the last fourteen years than methods of female contraception in the last seventy. That's disappointing, but not surprising. Of reviews for contraception that we've collected at The Lowdown, over 80 per cent are for five contraceptive methods that were developed over three decades ago.

The alternative hormonal contraceptives to the pill have benefits that can be used to your advantage. Firstly, if preventing pregnancy is your priority, they are incredibly effective and you don't have to remember to use them every day. These methods can lighten or stop your periods and some options, such as the hormonal coil, use very low hormone levels if you are wary about hormonal side effects. We look at other health benefits of different contraceptives in Chapter 4.

Currently, *all* hormonal methods of contraception are intended for use by those with a uterus. Given this bias, it may then seem like contraception is primarily a 'woman's issue' – although not everyone who uses contraception will identify as a woman – with the onus on us to prevent pregnancy as best we can. In truth, contraception should be *everyone's* responsibility, but there's still a lot of unravelling of expectations and cultural norms to get there.

Will we be seeing men taking greater ownership of their reproductive health in the future? In Chapter 12, we look at what might lie ahead for male contraceptives.

## You do you

Contraception, and in particular hormonal contraception, is one of those areas of health that sparks a lot of debate. Some may be evangelical about one method; others might view it more as a medieval torture device – no one will have the exact same experience. We all have different comfort zones and tolerances; for example, some might see the discomfort or pain of a coil fitting as worth it for the years that follow, when they don't have to think about contraception at all. In fact, The Lowdown's founder Alice only mustered up the courage to get her copper coil (IUD) fitted after suffering for years from the side effects of her contraceptive pill. It's all relative, and often what you've experienced before can impact your confidence to try another method. But there's no rhyme or reason with hormones, and your side effects from one method don't predict the side effects you'll experience from another.

It's an emotional decision as well as a physical one. Experiences and side effects are nuanced and it can be difficult to predict how an individual might feel on one type of hormonal contraception, particularly if it's their first experience with contraception. There is no one-size-fits-all solution, and similarly, encounters can vary for an individual depending on their stage of life, so the type of contraception that felt good in your twenties may end up not suiting you in your thirties. So, being informed, while keeping an open mind, can be the best way to approach making this decision.

## Hormonal contraception, but not the pill

We've found that a lot of people don't know that all hormonal contraceptives contain the same ingredients as contraceptive pills, they're just put into our bodies in different ways. As with the pill, other types of hormonal contraception work to prevent pregnancy by making the fluid in the cervix thicker (and less sperm friendly), preventing the lining of the uterus from becoming thick enough to host a fertilised egg, and some will also prevent ovulation. For anyone seeking alternatives to the pill, popular options include the hormonal coil, implant, injection, patch or vaginal ring.

The hormonal options covered in this chapter have all followed on the heels of the pill as derivatives of it and work in a similar way, but are more or less invasive in terms of how they're fitted and have varying pros and cons.

## Methods of contraception: your cheat sheet

| Type | Hormones | Method | Brands |
|---|---|---|---|
| Hormonal | Progestogen | Progestogen-only pill | See page 37 |
| | | Hormonal coil (IUS) | Mirena, Levosert, Benilexa, Kyleena, Jaydess |
| | | Implant | Nexplanon |
| | | Injection | Depo-Provera, Sayana Press, Noristerat |
| | Progestogen and oestrogen ('combined methods') | Combined pill | See page 36 |
| | | Patch | Evra |
| | | Vaginal ring | NuvaRing, SyreniRing |
| Non-hormonal | No hormones | Copper coil (IUD) | Brands include the Nova-T, Neo-Safe, T-Safe, Copper T380 and Flexi-T. (The Ballerine IUB and GyneFix are similar to the IUD.) |
| | | Fertility awareness methods (FAM) | This umbrella term includes methods like the symptothermal method and breastfeeding (Lactational Amenorrhea Methods (LAM)) |
| | | Digital contraception | Natural Cycles |
| | | Barrier methods | Male condom, female condom, cap, diaphragm |
| | | Permanent methods | Vasectomy (male sterilisation), female sterilisation (tubal occlusion) |

## Progestogen-only hormonal contraception

Just like the progestogen-only pill, the following methods only contain progestogen. This makes them ideal for anyone who has been told that they can't use combined hormonal contraception. These methods are referred to as LARCs, which stands for long-acting reversible contraception. Essentially, you can 'set it and forget', ditching the daily pill reminders. UK statistics show that demand for LARCs has gone up since 2019, with 36 per cent of women under twenty-five and 53 per cent of women over twenty-five using a type of LARC as their main method of contraception in 2022–2023.[1]

### The hormonal coil (IUS)

Over 99 per cent effective with perfect and typical use.[2]

Overall satisfaction rating: ★★★☆☆ 3.5/5 from 566 reviews

As rated by users at thelowdown.com

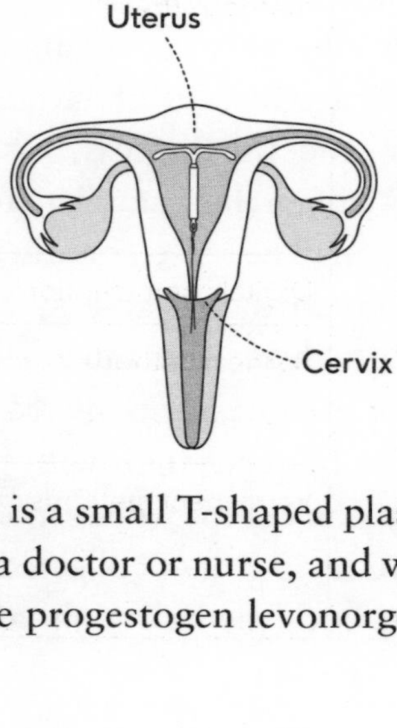


The hormonal coil is a small T-shaped plastic device inserted into the uterus by a doctor or nurse, and works by delivering a small dose of the progestogen levonorgestrel directly into the uterus. The acronym IUS stands for intrauterine system, which is interchangeably used with IUD, which stands for intrauterine device, often depending on where you are in the world. In the UK, healthcare professionals now use the term LNG-IUD (meaning levonorgestrel intrauterine device) to describe the hormonal coil. It's over 99 per cent effective and can be used as contraception for anywhere between three and eight years, depending on which brand you choose.

There are currently five types of hormonal coil available in the UK (see opposite). The three 'standard' coils containing 52 mg of the progestogen levonorgestrel are the Mirena, Levosert and Benilexa. The Mirena, Levosert and Benilexa are licensed for eight years for contraception.[3] These brands stop ovulation in around 25 per cent of women in the first year of use, so many women still experience monthly cyclical symptoms, but they are also amazing at lightening or stopping periods. If you were using one of these coils a few years ago you would have been told it 'ran out' after five years and would have had to have it replaced. However, more recent studies looking at what happens to pregnancy rates in years six, seven and eight after having these coils fitted show the coils maintain their effectiveness during this time.[4]

Two smaller coils are also available: the Kyleena, which lasts for five years, and the Jaydess, which lasts for three years. Because they are slightly smaller in size, they may be more comfortable to fit. They also contain lower doses of progestogen than the standard coils so may have fewer or lesser side effects, although there isn't much evidence to support this. Due to the low level of hormone, bleeds may not be as light or may be more frequent than with the other coils, and in most people they don't stop ovulation.

The contraceptive review data collected on The Lowdown website tells us that both the hormonal and copper coils are

## Hormonal coil brands

| | Mirena | Levosert | Benilexa | Kyleena | Jaydess |
|---|---|---|---|---|---|
| Size (W x H) | 32 x 32 mm | 32 x 32 mm | 32 x 32 mm | 28 x 30 mm | 29 x 30 mm |
| Size of inserter tube | 4.4 mm | 4.8 mm | 4.8 mm | 3.8 mm | 3.8 mm |
| Licensed length of use | 8 years OR 10 years if over 45 | 8 years OR 10 years if over 45 | 8 years OR 10 years if over 45 | 5 years | 3 years |
| Initial dose of levonorgestrel hormone released every 24 hours | 20 mcg | 20.1 mcg | 20.1 mcg | 17.5 mcg | 14 mcg |

among the highest-rated methods for overall satisfaction on our site. Once fitted 57–60 per cent of women reported their coils being 'very good' or 'excellent', over double the proportion that reported the same for the combined or progestogen-only pill.[5]

*Getting a coil fitted*

Before your coil is fitted, your GP or healthcare professional will have a short consultation with you and may ask you to do a pregnancy test. Often there will be an assistant in the room to help your doctor or nurse make sure they have everything they need, and to chat with you and help you during the procedure.

Your doctor or nurse will then examine inside your vagina to see the size and position of your uterus, and use a speculum to see the cervix (the neck of the uterus at the top of the vagina) by holding the walls of the vagina open. Local anaesthetic can be used at this point to numb the cervix and make the coil-fitting procedure less uncomfortable. Once the local anaesthetic has had time to work, your doctor or nurse will use an instrument called a tenaculum to hold the cervix so they can insert a slim plastic measuring device called a sound in order to measure the length of the uterus. Following this, the coil can be inserted into the uterus. The tube used to insert the coil is removed and the coil is left in place. The coil has two threads that hang through the neck of the uterus into the vagina which your doctor or nurse may trim for comfort.

It is important to be aware that all procedures like this can trigger what is known medically as a 'vasovagal response'. This means your heart rate and blood pressure drop and you may feel nauseous, light-headed and even faint. If you feel like this, your doctor or nurse may check your heart rate and blood pressure. These symptoms shouldn't last long, and your

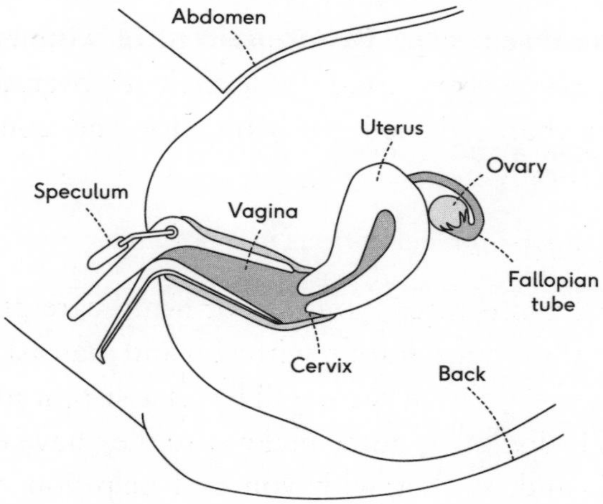


healthcare professional will be trained in how to manage this.

By now you'll know our mantra: everyone's different. This goes for how uncomfortable or painful you may find the fitting experience, too. On the day of your fitting, wear loose, comfortable clothes that are easy to change in and out of. Some clinics may recommend taking painkillers such as paracetamol or ibuprofen an hour before your fitting, and to continue these as instructed on the packet for as long as the discomfort lasts. Despite being widely advised, there's actually no evidence that taking painkillers before a fitting significantly helps reduce pain during an insertion. Guidelines in the UK now recommend everyone should be offered pain relief at their fitting.[6] The options such as a local anaesthetic spray, gel or injection can be discussed with the doctor or nurse during the coil-fitting appointment, or beforehand if you're offered a pre-fitting consultation. However, depending on the availability or staff training for services in your area, not all methods of pain relief, particularly injections, are always available. It's unfortunately a bit of a postcode lottery.

## The Lowdown's coil fitting pain relief cheat sheet

### Before your appointment

- Discuss pain relief options in a pre-fitting appointment, or over the phone to the clinic or GP practice. This is also a good opportunity to talk through any other anxieties you have about the procedure.
- Your doctor or nurse will consider your medical history and be able to advise what pain relief they have available.
- Clinical guidance now states that everyone should be offered adequate pain relief for a coil fitting.

### What pain relief options can you ask about?

- Depending on availability, you can request a local anaesthetic injection to the cervix, or a numbing spray or cream, with the spray being the most common option.
- Fewer places may offer anaesthetic injections, as they can come with risks like an allergic reaction, so require more equipment and more training for clinicians.
- Most places usually have access to numbing sprays. If they aren't able to offer any local anaesthetic, it's OK to discuss whether you'd like to go ahead with the fitting at all.

### On the day

- Some people like to take paracetamol and/or ibuprofen an hour before their procedure. Although there's no evidence it helps pain during the fitting, it does help cramps afterwards.[7]

- If you forgot to ask about pain relief, or didn't have a pre-fitting consultation, you can still discuss the above pain relief at any point up until the procedure starts.
- If you have numbing spray or cream, it will be applied to the cervix and takes a few minutes to work. The effect will wear off after an hour or so.
- If you have the anaesthetic injection, it is injected into your cervix, which can hurt a bit in itself. It too can take a few minutes to work and will wear off after a few hours.
- 'Vocal local' is a phrase that medics use, meaning that a relaxed environment with a chatty, distracting assistant is also useful as part of pain relief. This is why it is so important that you feel comfortable, in control and trust the person doing your procedure – as this has the ability to reduce the discomfort you may feel.

### If you're in pain

- Always tell the person doing your fitting if you're in pain, and if you feel it's becoming too much. They will be monitoring you throughout the fitting.
- If needed, the procedure can be stopped and you can discuss the best course of action.
- It's normal to have some cramping for a few hours after your coil has been inserted. Hot-water bottles and simple painkillers like paracetamol or ibuprofen can help. You may experience some mild cramping pain on and off in the first few weeks after having the coil inserted too.

- If you have pain that isn't controlled with paracetamol and ibuprofen, or you have other symptoms like abnormal bleeding, vaginal discharge or a fever, speak to a healthcare professional.

If your hormonal coil is fitted in the first five days of your cycle, you'll be protected immediately against pregnancy, but if it's fitted after that point in your cycle, you'll need to use another form of contraception for seven days. FYI, you can have your coil fitted during your period. If you switched from another contraceptive method, whether you need to use condoms for seven days after fitting will depend on the type of contraception you were using, if you were using it reliably and if you've had sex in the last seven days, so discuss this with your healthcare professional.

---

**Q:** Is it safe to use a menstrual cup with an IUD?

**A:** There hasn't been a large number of research studies looking at coil and menstrual cup use, but some evidence suggests there might be a slightly increased risk of your coil coming out while using a menstrual cup.[8]

You should follow the manufacturer's instructions for your menstrual cup, but generally they should sit low in the vagina and should form a light seal with the vaginal walls. The seal should be broken and any suction released before removing a menstrual cup and take care not to accidentally pull on the coil threads when doing so. Check your threads regularly and always after using a menstrual cup.

---

*Checking your coil threads*

Once you've had the coil fitted. you should check the threads four weeks after. This is important in order to check if your coil has fallen out (expulsion) or moved. Doctors used to get everybody to return for an examination four to six weeks after a fitting, but now self-checks are recommended because it's easy, you don't have to miss work and, well, COVID happened.

Expulsion can happen in up to one in twenty women, most commonly within the first three months after fitting, or sometimes up to a year.[9] The coil can also move down into the cervix, known as partial expulsion, lessening its contraceptive effect, and even perforate (make a hole in) the wall of the uterus. Perforation is rare but can happen in about one in one thousand coil fittings. Feeling your coil threads is therefore a really important way to check in with your coil and get to know your body. As the most common time for a coil to come out is within the first three months after fitting and after a period, it's recommended to check your threads every four weeks. Some practitioners relax the four-week rule after the first three months but will still recommend self-checks at regular intervals.

To self-check that the coil is still in place, feel for the two thin threads hanging down through the cervix at the top of the vagina. With your fingers inside the vagina, you should be able to feel your cervix, which is smooth and firm, and feels just like the tip of your nose. You may not be able to easily identify two separate threads, and that's fine. They soften over time and can end up feeling a bit like dental floss. If you can't feel them at all, don't panic, this is also pretty normal but you should contact your GP or local sexual health service for a check-up.

Before you are seen, your clinician will discuss whether

you might need emergency contraception and advise you to use another form of contraception until you can be examined to check the coil threads. When you are examined, the clinician will use a speculum to hold the vaginal walls open in order to look for your threads and check for any other problems. If the threads can't be seen, your clinician may be able to find them and pull them back down using a device called a thread retriever. If this isn't possible, the next step is to arrange an ultrasound and provide you with different contraception to keep you protected from pregnancy. If the ultrasound shows the coil isn't in the right position, your healthcare professional will discuss the next steps for removal or replacement of the coil. If the coil is confirmed to be in the correct position you can continue to use it for contraception.

---

**Q:** Will my partner be able to feel my coil strings during sex?

**A:** While it is entirely possible to feel these strings, it is more likely than not your partner won't feel anything at all. A Lowdown poll of 1,372 users determined that 29 per cent of partners have felt the coil during sex, while 71 per cent of partners have not.[10] However, feeling the coil during sex doesn't necessarily mean it's painful. A study in 2017 determined that only 3–9 per cent of partners have experienced enough discomfort from the coil strings to cause them to discontinue sex. The threads may tickle or occasionally nudge the tip of a penis, especially soon after insertion. However, the threads tend to soften over time reducing this feeling.[11]

---

## The implant

Over 99 per cent effective with perfect and typical use.[12]

Overall satisfaction rating: ★★★☆☆ 2.8/5 from 584 reviews

As rated by users at thelowdown.com

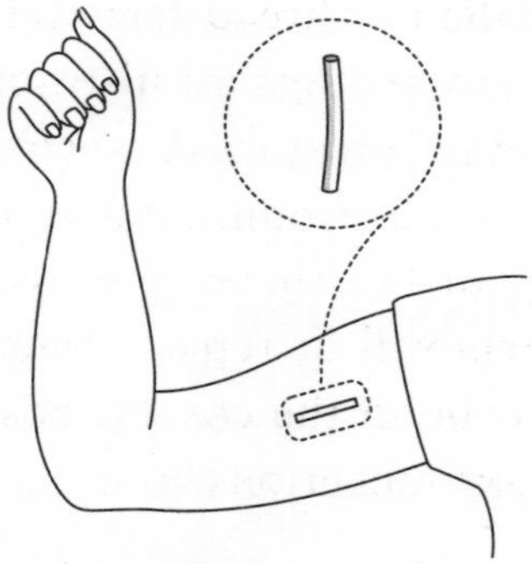

Implant

The implant contains a progestin called etonorgestrel, which is very similar to desogestrel found in the progestogen-only pill. Having an implant inserted is usually a super-quick procedure performed by a doctor or nurse. A small flexible plastic rod, about the size of a matchstick, is inserted under the skin in the upper arm (which is numbed using local anaesthetic), and kept in place for three years, after which it needs to be replaced or removed. Unlike other contraceptives, there's only one brand of implant available in the UK: Nexplanon. In other parts of the world, a brand called Jadelle is used, which uses two small plastic rods instead of one, and can be inserted for up to five years.

At over 99 per cent effective, the implant is the most effective method of contraception and technically more effective than a vasectomy – a permanent method of contraception known as male sterilisation (more on this later on).

The implant is also thought to be more effective than other methods like the coil because, as we've seen, IUDs come with the small risk of either expulsion or not sitting in quite the right position in the uterus after fitting, which you don't get with the implant. Once fitted, you will be able to feel the implant just underneath the skin. Rarely the implant can move so if you can no longer feel it, your doctor or nurse will need to check this, sometimes with an ultrasound scan (more on this in Chapter 6).

The implant can be fitted any time during your cycle; if fitted in the first five days of your cycle you'll be protected from pregnancy immediately, at any other times, you'll need to wait to have sex or use condoms for seven days. Some medications make the implant less effective, so speak to your doctor if this is relevant to you, as an alternative contraceptive may be required.

## The injection

Over 99 per cent effective with perfect use; around 94–98 per cent effective with typical use.[13]

Overall satisfaction rating: ★★★☆☆ 2.9/5 from 269 reviews

As rated by users at thelowdown.com

The contraceptive injection is another LARC method that's super effective at preventing pregnancy. There are two main types in the UK, which both contain the progestogen medroxyprogesterone acetate:

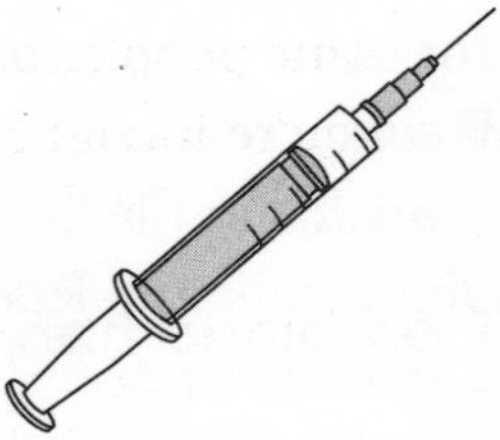

Injection

- **The Depo-Provera injection** is the most commonly prescribed in the UK. It lasts for thirteen weeks, and is injected by a healthcare professional into the muscle, usually in your buttock.
- **The Sayana Press injection** contains the same type of progestogen and lasts the same amount of time as the

Depo-Provera, but once a healthcare professional has shown you how, you can inject yourself at home into the skin at the top front of your thigh, or fleshy bit of your abdomen.

The Noristerat injection is not commonly prescribed in the UK or US any more, but it's still used in Europe, Africa and South America. It contains a different type of progestogen to the other two types, needs to be injected by a healthcare professional, and is only effective for up to eight weeks.

You can start the injection at any time during your menstrual cycle. If you have it within the first five days of your cycle, you will be protected from pregnancy straight away. Any other time in your cycle, and you'll need to use condoms for seven days before it is effective. Once the injection has been given, it can't be removed or stopped before the expiry date, which could be a downside if you're experiencing unwanted side effects.

It's the only method of contraception that has been shown to impact return of fertility after stopping in the short term for some people, but we'll get into this later (jump to Chapter 9 if you're intrigued).

## Combined hormonal contraception

Moving on to combined hormonal methods of contraception other than the pill: the patch and the vaginal ring. These methods work in the exact same way as the combined pill. They contain both synthetic oestrogen and progestogen; it's just a different way of getting these hormones into your body. And just as you can run your combined pill packets together to take continuously without a break to skip your withdrawal bleed (i.e. the 'fake' period you get when using hormonal contraception), you can do the same with these methods. Let's get into it.

## The patch

Around 99 per cent effective with perfect use; around 91–93 per cent effective with typical use.[14]

Overall satisfaction rating: ★★★☆☆ 3.5/5 from 101 reviews

As rated by users at thelowdown.com

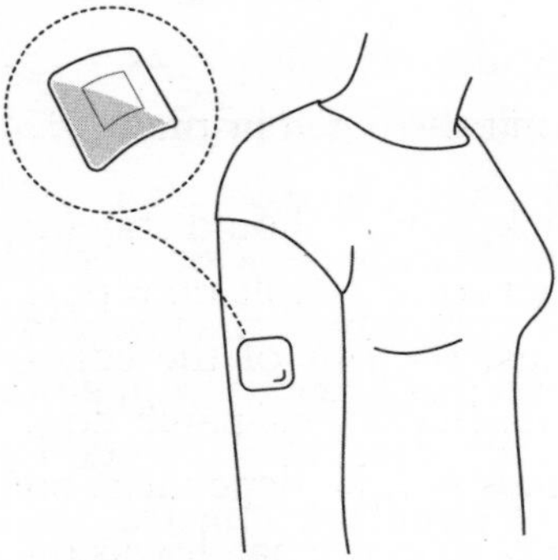

Patch

The patch offers lots of the benefits of the combined pill but without the need to remember to take it daily. You change your patch on the same day each week for three weeks, then have the option to have a patch-free break of four to seven days, where you will likely have a withdrawal bleed. After the patch-free break, a new patch should be applied (even if you're still bleeding). It's fine to skip it altogether to avoid bleeding by putting on a new patch every week. You may see in some leaflets, or hear from pharmacists, that the patch is less effective if you weigh over 90 kg and to try an alternative method. This is based on limited research evidence[15] and does not mean you cannot use it at all, but extra precautions such as condoms would be recommended. It works immediately if you start using the patch in the first five days of your period, or you can start at any point in your cycle and use condoms for seven days.

Currently, the patch only comes in a pale beige colour, which is sorely disappointing. This means it's much less discreet for anyone who uses it that isn't white. The lack of skin tone options for the contraceptive patch is just another example of how Black women and women of colour continue to be let down and overlooked by the healthcare system. If you'd like to show your support to change this, at the time of writing, Reproductive Justice Initiative have founded the Clap Back on the Contraceptive Patch campaign (see website in Resources) which you're able to sign up to digitally.

---

**Q:** I love swimming and exercising, won't the patch just fall off?

**A:** The contraceptive patch is super sticky and it should stay on during a bath, shower or swimming, but some people do report having issues with them sticking. If just the tips of the edges are coming off, you should be protected. But if your patch does make a break for it, then your next steps will be dependent on how long it's been off for and how many days the patch was on before it came off, so check the instructions.

---

## The vaginal ring

Around 99 per cent effective with perfect use; around 91–93 per cent effective with typical use.[16]

**Overall satisfaction rating:** ★★★★☆ **3.7**/5 from 48 reviews

As rated by users at thelowdown.com

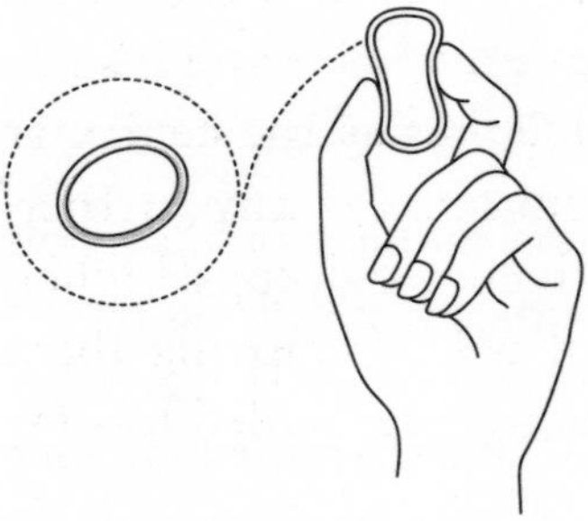

**Vaginal ring**

This is the contraceptive that stumps a lot of people when you show them a picture. The vaginal ring is a soft, flexible plastic ring that's about 5 cm in diameter. It sort of looks like a glow stick before you've snapped it to become fluorescent, or a big plastic hairband. It has the same effectiveness rating as the combined pill and the patch. You insert it into the vagina for three weeks (twenty-one days), then either choose to have a seven-day ring-free break, which as with the patch you can shorten to four days, or just pop a new one in to skip your bleed. We asked 1,976 people about whether they'd use the vaginal ring if they knew more about it, and 68 per cent said yes.[17]

The ring can be a bit fiddly to insert and get used to but, with practice, you'll soon be an expert.

- First things first, wash your hands.
- Squeeze the ring between your thumb and finger so the two edges you're holding on to are pretty much touching.
- Gently insert it into your vagina and push in until it

feels comfortable and secure, similar to how a tampon feels.

- To remove it, gently hook a finger under one edge of the ring and pull it out. When you're done with one ring remember to bin it, never flush it.

The ring should stay pinched together inside you, just as you inserted it. Unlike a cap or diaphragm, the ring does not need to cover the entrance to the uterus to work. But it should be far enough inside that you can't feel it and it's not uncomfortable. It can't get lost inside you as the cervix at the top of the vagina prevents it from moving any further. You can safely use tampons[18] and menstrual cups[19] when your ring is inserted, just be careful when removing them so that the ring doesn't come out too, or get pulled too far out of place.

You can start using the ring at any time during your menstrual cycle. If you insert it on the first five days of your cycle, you will be protected from pregnancy right away. If you insert it at any other time in your cycle then you will need to use condoms or avoid sex for seven days.

---

**Q:** Do you take the ring out during sex, or keep it in?

**A:** The vaginal ring is designed to be kept in during sex. You and your partner may or may not be able to feel it, but most people don't find it bothersome. If you choose to take it out for sex, wash the ring with warm water and pop it back in. It will still protect you from pregnancy if it's reinserted within three hours.[20]

---

## Non-hormonal contraceptives

In recent years, we've seen a shift in contraception preferences, and people are increasingly interested in non-hormonal methods. At the time of writing, 21 per cent of women who had used The Lowdown's contraception recommender tool told us that they were not open to using hormones.[21]

Non-hormonal contraception might suit your needs for lots of different reasons. For example, if you're not able to use certain hormonal contraceptives due to your medical history, current medication or medical conditions. Perhaps access to hormonal contraception isn't so easy or your sex life is on the more occasional side. However, some require close day-to-day monitoring, so might not be as suited to your schedule or lifestyle.

### The copper coil (IUD)

Over 99 per cent effective with perfect and typical use.[22]

Overall satisfaction rating: ★★★½☆ **3.5**/5 from 566 reviews

As rated by users at thelowdown.com

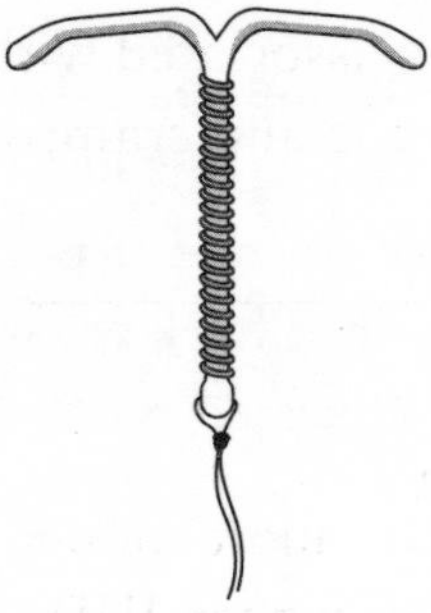

**Copper coil**

The copper coil (IUD) is the non-hormonal cousin of the hormonal IUS. It's a small T-shaped plastic device wrapped in copper wire and inserted by a doctor or nurse. Just like its cousin, it's over 99 per cent effective. It can be used as contraception for anywhere between five to ten years, depending on which brand you choose. The copper coil is the only LARC available for anyone who wants to try out non-hormonal contraception but doesn't want to have to remember to use it every day or every time you have sex. Because the risk of pregnancy is so small, it's so low maintenance *and* it doesn't contain hormones, we've seen an uptake of people wanting to try the copper coil over recent years. In fact, UK statistics show that copper coil use is up from 4 per cent in 2012–2013 to 10 per cent in 2022–2023.[23]

But … how does copper prevent pregnancy? Essentially copper is toxic to eggs and sperm. It affects how well sperm can swim, and stops them from reaching or even surviving to meet an egg before they can fertilise it. In the rare event that any sperm do survive and reach an egg, the copper coil also causes a very mild inflammatory reaction in the lining of the uterus so the fertilised egg can't implant. This clever bit of science is also the reason why the copper coil works as soon as it is inserted, and can be fitted up to five days after sex or five days after your estimated ovulation date as emergency contraception (more on this in Chapter 8).

While the copper coil is zapping any sperm, The Lowdown's review data at the time of writing shows that 76 per cent of users reported they experienced period-like cramps, 41 per cent reported lower back pain and 69 per cent said they had heavier periods.[24] We'll get into these kinds of side effects in more detail in Chapter 5, but it seems the main toss-up to this method is choosing between fewer side effects associated with hormones, in place of potentially heavier bleeds and cramps.

**New coils, who dis?**

The copper and hormonal coils have two more non-hormonal intrauterine cousins: the Gynefix copper IUD and the IUB Ballerine. Both are over 99 per cent effective and can be used for up to five years. The idea behind these methods is that because they don't follow the traditional T-shape of other IUDs they may be less painful to insert or sit better in the uterus. The Gynefix is a tube of copper wrapped around a plastic thread, while the IUB Ballerine consists of seventeen copper pearls on a sphere-shaped metal frame. These aren't widely available in the UK at the time of writing, and they're very new methods in general, so our insight on how people get on with these methods is limited, as is research on rates of expulsion.

---

**Q:** Can I have an IUD if I've never given birth vaginally before?

**A:** Yes, you can. Coil fitters are very comfortable inserting coils in women of all ages who have or have not given birth. Some women may find coil insertions easier after giving birth as the hole in the cervix known as the 'os' (the entrance to the uterus) will be bigger, but others may find scar tissue or changes after birth can make it more challenging. So if you have given birth vaginally before, you should be offered pain relief for a coil fitting – everyone should have the option of good pain relief.

---

### Fertility awareness methods (FAM)

Estimates of effectiveness vary from 76 per cent with typical use to over 99 per cent with perfect use.[25]

Overall satisfaction rating: ★★★★☆ 4.3/5 from 154 reviews

As rated by users at thelowdown.com

Fertility awareness methods (FAM), a modern form of the 'rhythm method', have been used in some way for thousands of years to prevent pregnancy. Fertility awareness is an umbrella term encompassing different ways of identifying your fertile window by keeping track of your menstrual cycle and other biological signs of ovulation. These methods (which include both digital and non-digital ways of tracking your fertility) are the highest-rated method of contraception on The Lowdown, with an average rating of 4.3 out of 5.[26]

FAM is another form of contraception that's been talked about a lot over recent years. We often hear from women who are ditching the pill to find out who they 'really' are without hormones and what their 'normal' menstrual cycle is like – either because they've been on hormonal contraception since their early teens or because they've been scared away from hormones due to the rise in contraception misinformation online. Anecdotally, we've had people tell us it can be like having a personality transplant due to no longer experiencing extreme mood swings from hormonal contraception. On the flip side, we hear from others who find themselves unexpectedly pregnant when using FAM. If used properly, these methods can be as effective as the pill. But unlike using the pill, there are more things for you to keep track of for this to be the case.

These methods require close attention to detail, dedication and discipline to use effectively, and there are a few, seemingly minor, things people can forget to consider while using FAM. Avoiding sex or using condoms when you're most fertile is key to avoiding an unplanned pregnancy, although condoms themselves have a typical failure rate of around 18 per cent. Some use condoms all the time for the first three to six months of starting FAM, while learning how to interpret indicators of ovulation. Lots of factors can affect how you interpret these indicators, such as illness, stress, lifestyle or travel, meaning your fertile window may not always be easy to accurately identify and can change from cycle to cycle. Let's get into what these fertile indicators look like with each type of FAM method.

*The symptothermal method*

After one year: over 99 per cent effective with perfect use; around 98 per cent with typical use.[27]

**Overall satisfaction rating:** ★★★★☆ **3.7**/5 from 8 reviews

As rated by users at thelowdown.com

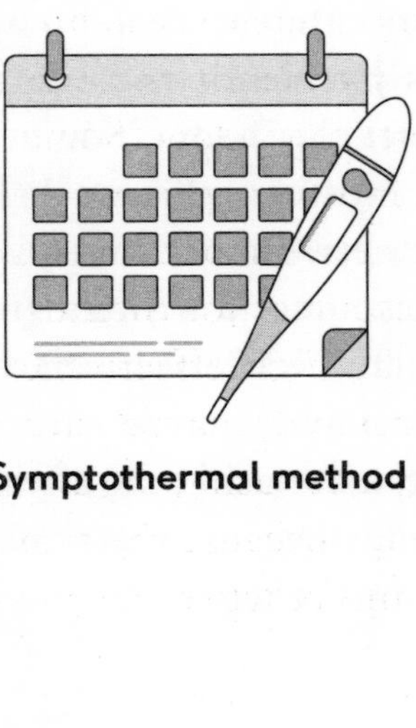

**Symptothermal method**

Basal body temperature (BBT) refers to your lowest natural body temperature recorded after resting. In 1906, Theodoor Hendrik van de Velde,[28] a Dutch gynaecologist, noticed a two-phase change in BBT in women during the menstrual cycle, with a small rise in BBT noticed after ovulation. This is due to progesterone levels increasing as you head towards your period. The symptothermal method pays close attention to indicators like waking BBT (measured first thing in the morning), as well as cervical fluid, cycle length and other signals from the body to identify when you ovulate. If you want to prevent pregnancy, don't have sex or make sure to use condoms in your fertile window, which is usually around six days, combining the day of ovulation, plus the days leading up to it that sperm can survive within the female body.

Generally, this method can be more difficult to use if your periods are considered irregular, because it can be harder to predict when you will ovulate. It's also probably not going to be a reliable method for you if you don't have a structured routine to monitor your symptoms. Even things like poor sleep and drinking alcohol can affect your BBT, so this is something to keep in mind. Fertility awareness practitioners or educators can teach you how to practise fertility awareness methods by identifying signs of ovulation and calculating your fertile window. Some practitioners work in NHS clinics but most are private. Fertility UK provides access to a UK-wide network of trained and accredited FAM practitioners (see Resources for their details).

Data shows similar high effectiveness rates for perfect use (over 99 per cent) and, maybe surprisingly, typical use (around 98 per cent) after using the symptothermal method for one year,[29] perhaps because the typical users are highly motivated to learn and practise this method. However, the level of motivation women and partners experience may change with time and circumstances.[30]

## Digital contraception

Natural Cycles is around 98 per cent effective with perfect use; around 93 per cent effective with typical use.[31]

**Overall satisfaction rating: ★★★★☆ 4.2/5 from 105 reviews**

As rated by users at thelowdown.com

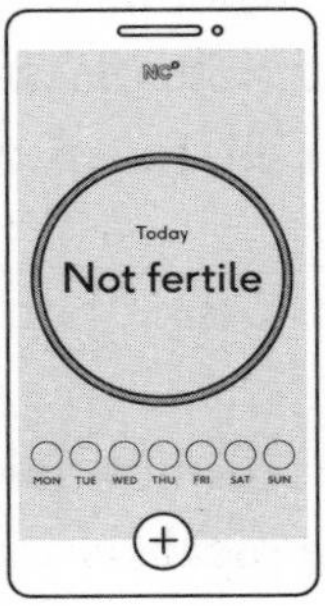


**Natural Cycles**

Digital contraception has been the biggest innovation in contraception in recent years. The only app currently cleared for use as a contraceptive in the UK is Natural Cycles. It uses an algorithm to calculate the days you're fertile, based on detecting and predicting ovulation from the information you give it each day, such as where you are in your cycle, waking temperature (based on BBT as described above) and optional luteinising hormone (LH) results from at-home urine-sample tests. To make the app easy to use, days where it is considered safe to have unprotected sex appear as 'green days', whereas 'red days' warn you that you are likely to be fertile and therefore may fall pregnant if you have unprotected sex. FYI, if you're using a period tracking app to track your cycle, you shouldn't rely on this alone for contraception as it doesn't take into account signs of ovulation to calculate your fertile window.

If you have irregular cycles or struggle to input data regularly it can make predicting ovulation with the app more difficult. As can things which affect your BBT, like feeling sick or hungover or sleeping differently. While this doesn't reduce the effectiveness of the app, it will increase the number of red days on which you have to abstain from sex or use condoms, and if you're experiencing mostly red days then the app isn't doing much for you. This is why our doctors wouldn't recommend Natural Cycles to an eighteen-year-old student with a menstrual cycle that is still being established, who is potentially going out on lots of late nights and experiencing hangovers!

Natural Cycles clinical studies have shown the app to be 93 per cent effective with typical use, and 98 per cent effective with perfect use (perfect use means not having unprotected sex on red fertile days, and if using condoms, using these consistently and correctly).[32] This effectiveness rating is also determined by the company's ongoing monitoring of effectiveness rates that they are required to do as an FDA (US Food and Drug Administration) approved medical device.

Natural Cycles typical use effectiveness rating is on a par with the combined and progestogen-only pills, the patch and the vaginal ring. With all of these methods, it is down to the user to make sure they are being as efficient and effective as possible – whether that's knowing what counts as a missed pill, when to change the patch or how to properly insert a vaginal ring. With Natural Cycles, you must abstain from sex on red days if you want to use the app perfectly, or if using condoms on red days make sure you use these consistently and correctly. With that in mind, if you are using condoms on red fertile days you are actually relying on the effectiveness of condoms (around 82 per cent with typical use) for your contraception. If you use a condom incorrectly, it breaks or you don't use a condom on red days, you should consider emergency contraception.

Our data at The Lowdown suggests that some women love the digital contraceptive app Natural Cycles (it's currently rated 4.2 out of 5 stars from 105 reviews).[33] Lowdown users who use Natural Cycles tell us they love not having side effects from contraception impacting their mood, skin or sex drive, for example, and really getting to learn about how their body works.

Unlike other contraceptives, there's no requirement to consult a healthcare professional before you start or stop using digital contraceptive apps. However, their importance and usage should not be overstated. For reference, Natural Cycles has had around three million registered users globally in the last ten years,[34] while UN figures suggest that the pill is used by over 150 million people. Given there are almost a billion people using contraception, it's still a drop in the ocean.[35] We shouldn't forget that when it comes to the companies who make digital contraceptive apps, it's the first time anyone has spent money actively marketing a contraceptive to an audience. Most hormonal contraceptives are prescription medicines, which pharmaceutical companies are prohibited from marketing to the public in the UK and Europe. So that's also why we feel like digital contraception is being talked about so much.

The majority of users who have rated digital contraception 1 star on The Lowdown have told us they fell pregnant, with some stating their app had trouble detecting their ovulation accurately. Studies have shown unintended pregnancies do occur while using Natural Cycles, but these results match up with the published effectiveness rates mentioned above, and it is important to remember no contraceptive method is 100 per cent effective.[36]

There's also a cost as you have to pay a monthly or yearly subscription, compared to other contraceptive methods which are free on the NHS. And while it is becoming easier to track indicators of ovulation with digital contraception, as digital wearables like the Oura Ring and newer versions of the Apple Watch can track your temperature and link to your Natural Cycles app for a more accurate reading, this additional cost is prohibitive for some. Digital contraceptive apps are definitely not right for everybody, but work really well for some individuals, which is the same principle for any contraceptive.

## Barrier methods

'Barrier methods' is the term used to describe contraceptives that are physical barriers to sperm reaching an egg. From the Ancient Egyptians apparently using a paste of honey and acacia leaves in the vagina as a makeshift cervical cap (ouch) and Ancient Greeks and Romans allegedly using olive oil to prevent conception, to those in sixteenth-century Europe creating condom-style 'coverings' from light fabrics or even animal innards and skins (an infection waiting to happen?) – folk had to get pretty creative in days of yore.[37]

Nowadays, we're spoilt for choice when it comes to effective barrier methods. Condoms are highly accessible and the method most of us can confidently say we were taught how to use in school sex ed classes. As we hear people talk about ditching hormonal contraception, more brands of condoms appear on the market, to suit a range of needs. It's not just the options of vegan, chemical-free and latex-free condoms that have expanded – it's who they're marketed to. More condom brands are appealing directly to women. It's great to have more choices, and we love seeing a surge of female-founded condom brands trying to dispel the 'condoms don't feel good' narrative.

## Male condoms (aka external condoms)

Around 98 per cent effective with perfect use; around 82–87 per cent effective with typical use.[38]

**Overall satisfaction rating: ★★★★☆ 4.1/5 from 65 reviews**

As rated by users at thelowdown.com

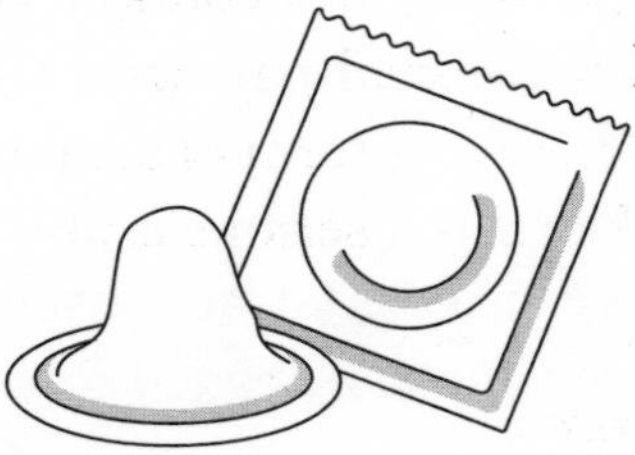

**Condom**

Fortunately, the days of wrapping a penis in sheep intestines are over. Condoms are made from thin latex or polyurethane sheets and come in a variety of sizes. They're worn on the penis to prevent sperm reaching the uterus after ejaculation. Before using, pinch the top to squeeze out any air, then roll down onto the penis. Once you've used it, discard it in the bin – it's a once-and-done situation. They're up to 98 per cent effective if used perfectly, easy to buy and use, hormone-free and with few, if any, side effects.

Potential hazards include having a condom break, split or slip off during sex, which is why choosing the correct size is important. If this happens, emergency contraception and an STI test should be considered. Oil-based lubricants can actually damage the latex in condoms, sometimes even causing them to break. So if you're using lube with a condom, make sure you pick a water- or silicon-based one. This is something that very few people know, but which to us, at least, feels like a Pretty Big

Deal. Plus, the effectiveness of condoms can also be impacted by vaginal medication for things like thrush, storing condoms in intense heat or cold, and using them past their expiry date. So it's best to store them away from direct sunlight, in a place where they won't easily get squashed, ripped or damaged.

Condoms are the only contraception that protect against STIs. Therefore, their usage should be considered essential unless you and your sexual partner are completely up-to-date with your sexual health checks. FYI, if your partner refuses to wear a condom or tries to talk you out of it because it doesn't feel good for them, this is a huge red flag to run for the hills. If it doesn't feel right, encourage your partner to try different sizes or brands which may improve pleasure. If a condom is removed without your consent (or your sexual partner pretends to put one on but doesn't do so), this is a form of sexual assault, sometimes called 'stealthing', and is a serious crime.

### Female condoms (aka internal condoms)

Around 95 per cent effective with perfect use; around 79 per cent effective with typical use.[39]

Overall satisfaction rating: ★★★☆☆ 3.5/5 from 4 reviews

As rated by users at thelowdown.com

Sometimes referred to as a Femidom, these are soft pouches made of a thin, strong plastic called polyurethane, nitrile or latex, that prevent pregnancy by stopping sperm from reaching the uterus and fertilising an egg. To use, squeeze the smaller ring at the closed end of the

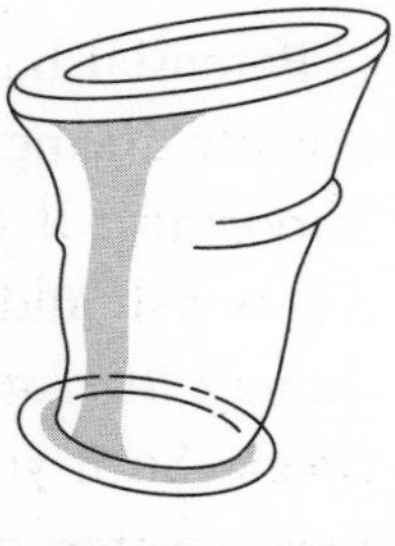

Female condom

condom and put it inside your vagina. Use your fingers to push the inner ring as far back into your vagina as you can, and then, with your fingers inside the condom, open the large ring at the open end of the condom – it should be outside the opening of the vagina. To remain effective, the penis must remain inside the condom. It's loose fitting and designed to move during sex, unlike a male condom. Remove the condom immediately after sex; gently pull it out and twist the large ring (this stops semen which is released after ejaculation from leaking out), then throw it in the bin.

Research shows that with typical use the female condom is around 79 per cent effective, while the male condom is around 82–87 per cent effective. With perfect use the male condom is 98 per cent effective, which is slightly more than the female condom at 95 per cent. Female condoms do also offer protection from STIs. Since The Lowdown's conception in 2019, and at the time of writing, there are only four reviews for this type of condom on our website.[40] While this isn't a proportional representation of the UK, it's a sure sign that this method really isn't widely used. Likely because it can be tricky to insert – if you're really prepared, you could insert it up to four hours before sex, but in reality, no one's doing that. It's also not as effective as male condoms, and not as easy to get your hands on, so the pros aren't really stacking in the female condom's favour.

### The cap or diaphragm

Cap: Around 78 per cent effective with perfect use and typical use.[41]
Diaphragm: Around 84–94 per cent effective with perfect use; 83–86 per cent effective with typical use.[42]

Overall satisfaction rating: ★★★★☆ 3.9/5 from 14 reviews

As rated by users at thelowdown.com

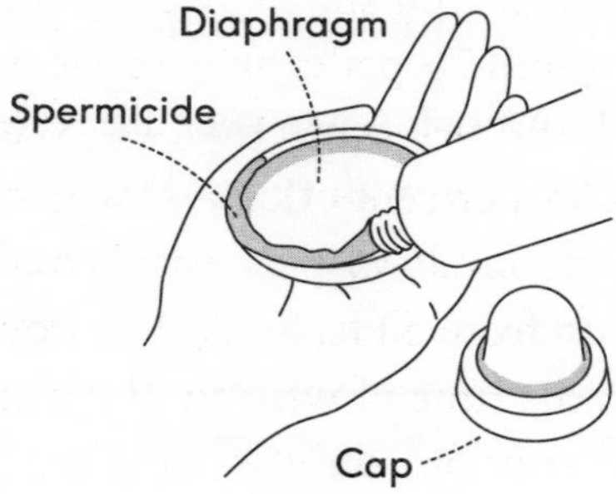

**Cap and diaphragm**

If you're looking for a more environmentally conscious option than a disposable condom, you could try a cap or diaphragm. They work by covering the cervix and stopping sperm from getting into the uterus. They're usually in the shape of a circular dome made of thin, soft silicone (although there are options of shapes, sizes and materials) that you insert into your vagina before sex. They should always be used with a gel that kills sperm, called spermicide, and placed in the vagina covering the cervix up to three hours before sex.[43] The effectiveness is user dependent, ranging from around 78 per cent up to 94 per cent effective with perfect use.

Both the cap and the diaphragm are reusable but must be left in place for a minimum of six hours after sex before being removed. Once removed it should be washed in warm water with a mild, unperfumed soap. You must not leave the diaphragm in for more than thirty hours or the cap for more than forty-eight hours.[44] You can buy a cap or diaphragm online, but it's best to have an in-person consultation with a healthcare professional in the first instance as they'll ensure they prescribe you the appropriate size and talk you through how to insert it. It can be a bit tricky to get the hang of, but some people love it. If you're a regular menstrual cup user, you'd probably get the hang of it pretty quickly. Again, it's not a widely reviewed method on The Lowdown in the UK, as it's a method that likely fell out of favour when newer hormonal methods were introduced with potentially less room for user error.

### The withdrawal method, aka the pull-out method

Around 96 per cent effective with perfect use; 80 per cent effective with typical use.[45]

Overall satisfaction rating: ★★★☆☆ 3.6/5 from 14 reviews

As rated by users at thelowdown.com

Some people dispute the use of the term 'contraceptive method' with this strategy, as its effectiveness is much lower than other methods, and timing is everything. A typical effectiveness of 80 per cent means 20 per cent of couples will get pregnant in a year. The chance of getting pregnant each month without any contraception is around 15–20 per cent, so you can see there's not much difference. The idea behind the withdrawal method relies on the penis being all the way out of the vagina before ejaculation and ejaculation occurring away from the vagina or vulva. This doesn't take into account issues with achieving this or the existence of pre-ejaculate (aka pre-cum).

Pre-cum is fluid that is discharged from a penis when it is aroused and usually occurs right before ejaculation. The fluid can act as a natural lubricant during sex. To quickly answer the question you've all been waiting for – *Can pre-cum cause pregnancy*? – the chances are very slim (touch wood, pun not intended). But if you don't want to get pregnant, it's best to avoid the risk. Pre-cum does not only occur in the moments just before orgasm. Some males might produce more pre-cum than others and at different times during sex. Many people also believe – and are told – that pre-cum does not contain any sperm. They are right but, before you get too excited, sperm has the potential to leak into pre-cum before it makes its way into the vagina. Sperm can linger in the penis after a previous ejaculation and mix with pre-cum while on its way out.

We know it's not a reliable method of contraception, but that doesn't mean people don't use it, or combine it with other methods. Doctors in the UK advise against the withdrawal method as a means of contraception on its own at *any* time during the menstrual cycle, but lots of people use it in addition to their usual contraceptive or alongside FAM methods, for example on their non-fertile days.

If you're going to do it, know the risks: 80 per cent effectiveness might sound quite high, but that's one in five couples using it who will get pregnant each year and compared to most other methods, it pales in comparison. Relying on the pull-out method can bring pregnancy paranoia each month too if your period is even a day or two late.

## Permanent contraception

OK, so what happens if you want to make the switch a little more ... permanent? If you know you don't want to have children, or have any more, this is where sterilisation might come in. The options are: for men, a vasectomy (aka 'the snip') and for women, female/tubal occlusion (aka having your 'tubes tied'). Having either can be a big decision and isn't one to be taken lightly. Because of this, at The Lowdown we've heard lots of stories of both men and women seeking sterilisation, but being refused by doctors with the words 'What if you change your mind?', or even, 'But what if you meet someone else?' So we'll preface this section by saying even though you may be sure you want sterilisation, it might take a while depending on waiting lists in your area.

### Vasectomy (male sterilisation)

Over 99 per cent effective with perfect and typical use.[46]

| Overall satisfaction rating: ★★★½☆ 3.6/5 from 7 reviews |
|---|

As rated by users at thelowdown.com

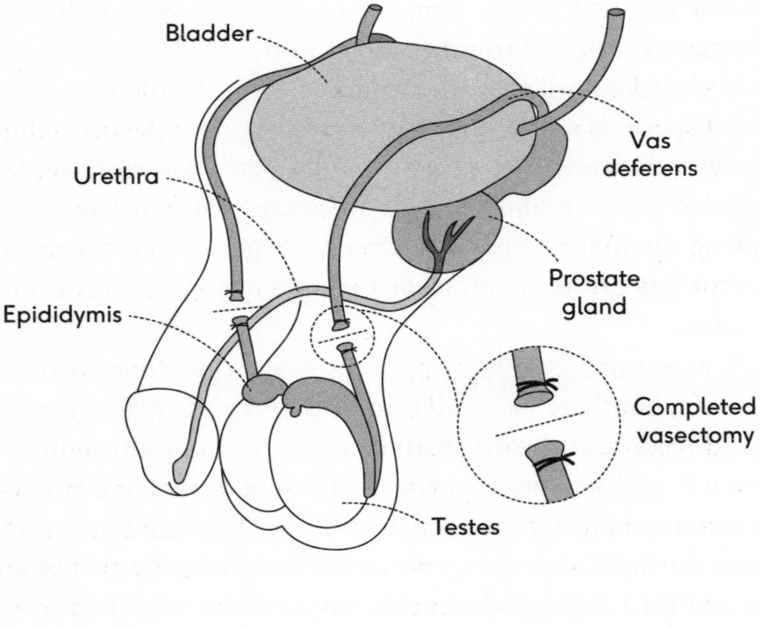

A vasectomy is a permanent surgical procedure that prevents pregnancy by cutting the vas deferens tubes (sperm ducts) which carry sperm from the testicles to the penis. This prevents the sperm from getting into semen (aka cum) which is the fluid that is ejaculated during sex. The surgery time is super-speedy, it's done under local anaesthetic (sometimes within a GP surgery or sexual health clinic) and side effects tend to be minor, usually some bruising and swelling of the scrotum (the sac that contains the testicles) that goes away within a couple of days of the procedure. If you're in the UK, getting a vasectomy is free on the NHS, but waiting lists can be long. It is possible to reverse a vasectomy, but it's not always guaranteed to work and it's more complicated than the original procedure. Plus, reversal is rarely funded by the NHS in the UK.

It can take several months for semen to be sperm-free after a vasectomy. Semen is tested after three months and at least twenty ejaculations to check whether sperm are still present and/or mobile.[47] If the sample suggests you could still cause pregnancy, you're recommended to re-test a sample every four to six weeks until the threshold to be non-fertile is reached. Or, if sperm is still present seven months after the procedure, the vasectomy is classed as a failure.[48] It's therefore recommended you use alternative contraception when having sex during the first few months after having a vasectomy until a doctor has given the all-clear that the procedure has been a success.

A vasectomy is over 99 per cent effective if done correctly. It's rare, but there's a small chance that the vas deferens tubes could reconnect due to small channels forming through scar tissue that allow sperm to wiggle through. Again, it's rare, but vasectomy failure could also just be down to human surgical error during a vasectomy procedure, and usually this would be identified through the initial semen testing described above.

**Q:** Given a vasectomy is one of the most straightforward ways to prevent pregnancy, why is the uptake so low?

We asked Dr Sophie Nicholls, a specialty doctor in sexual and reproductive health who has performed thousands of vasectomies, what she thinks . . .

**A:** 'Although I believe that the uptake of vasectomies is actually increasing, there are probably several reasons why vasectomy is not as common as other methods of contraception yet.

'Firstly, men have little to choose from when it comes to contraceptive options – from the slightly 'hit and miss' condom to the rather permanent thought of a vasectomy. Sometimes by the time they think about this latter option then their other halves already have their contraception sorted and it's only when their partners start to have issues or decide enough is enough that they are nudged in the direction of contemplating a vasectomy.

'I think the other reason vasectomies are less common is because men, unlike women, don't talk about these things so much between themselves, so some men may not be aware that this is potentially a good option for them. Some men don't think contraception is something they need to be responsible for, despite being fertile every day of the year. Others may be terrified of the thought of having a procedure in such a sensitive and embarrassing part of their body.

'We need to increase discussion about vasectomies amongst men, and women, to raise awareness, allay any fears and dispel myths around the procedure, and highlight this as a potential perfect option for those men who know they don't want to father any children in the future.'

### Female sterilisation (tubal occlusion)

Over 99 per cent effective with perfect and typical use.[49]

| |
|---|
| Overall satisfaction rating: ★★★★☆ 4.4/5 from 7 reviews |

As rated by users at thelowdown.com

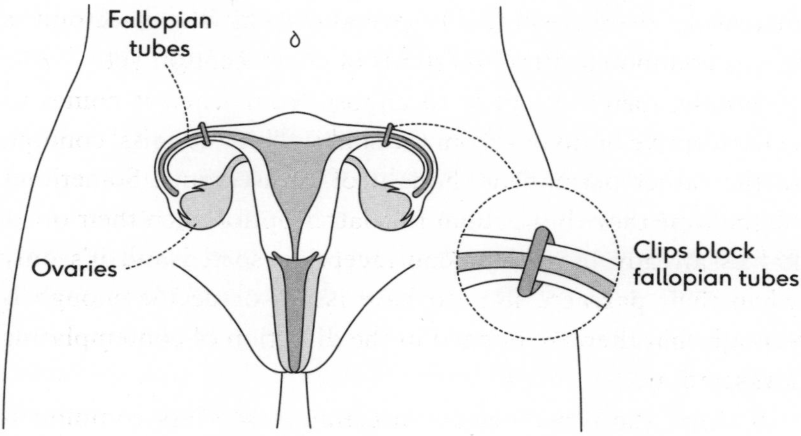


This is a permanent method to prevent pregnancy and it is not easily reversible. It involves a surgical procedure under anaesthetic that blocks or seals the fallopian tubes, usually using tiny clamps, to prevent eggs reaching sperm and becoming fertilised. While this does prevent pregnancy, your menstrual cycle will not be affected so you'll still ovulate and have periods. The recovery time can vary, depending on your general health and whether the procedure was done under local or general anaesthetic. Normally there's a bit of discomfort, which eases with a few days of rest. Sometimes, sterilisation can be done at the same time as a planned caesarean section (C-section). You'll need to use contraception until the day of the operation, and for at least seven days afterwards to avoid pregnancy (although not if it's done at the same time as a C-section).

In order to access sterilisation, you'll usually need to discuss it in detail with your GP – they will ask you a number of questions around your circumstances and may offer you counselling to help you decide. They'll likely also run through other types of LARC such as the implant, injection or coil. The implant is actually slightly more effective at preventing pregnancy (both over 99 per cent), as very rarely sterilisation can fail due to surgical error or sometimes the tubes rejoining.[50]

Currently in the UK, NHS hospitals are more likely to carry out sterilisation on women who are over thirty years old, and are less likely to want to perform this procedure if you do not have children. Anecdotally, lots of our Lowdown community told us they have faced backlash from doctors when asking for sterilisation even if they already have children. In a society where more people are child free by choice, why is our healthcare system sometimes reluctant to perform permanent methods of contraception, especially on women? This could be due to waiting times and the risk of surgery that requires a general anaesthetic, compared to relatively safe and inexpensive LARCs like the implant or coils. We often hear of people seeking private treatment as they haven't been able to get a referral for NHS-funded surgery in the UK when they wanted it.

# 4

# Contraception and your reproductive health

Often, when we think about contraception, it's as a way of preventing pregnancy: contra (against), conception (to get pregnant). But for many, its protection against pregnancy is secondary to its use as a type of medication to help manage conditions or symptoms. Hormonal contraception can be a go-to for doctors to treat a variety of issues, from managing premenstrual syndrome (PMS) or heavy or painful periods, to acne. It's also commonly used as a treatment option for conditions like polycystic ovary syndrome (PCOS) and endometriosis – we highlight these later in the chapter, to consider how contraception can help manage symptoms for both. We'll also explore what else can be done when hormonal contraception isn't an option.

Side effects from hormonal contraception get a lot of bad press (hello, mood swings). But when it successfully alleviates symptoms that can be so debilitating that they impede basic responsibilities like going to work, it's good to remember that not all side effects are awful. For instance, if we hadn't discovered that sildenafil, a drug first developed to treat heart problems like angina (chest pains due to reduced blood flow to the heart), was significantly more effective at causing erections than at relieving angina, then we wouldn't have Viagra!

Some of the most common reasons, other than preventing pregnancy, that GPs prescribe hormonal contraception include:

- Improving bleeding regularity and flow, often making periods lighter and more predictable.
- Stopping periods altogether, which can be especially beneficial to those who suffer with heavy bleeding and/or pain, for example due to fibroids.
- Premenstrual syndrome (PMS) and premenstrual dysphoric disorder (PMDD).
- Acne.
- Polycystic ovary syndrome (PCOS).
- Endometriosis.
- Adenomyosis.

## How to manage heavy or painful periods

If you have periods you will have around 450 on average in your lifetime.[1] That's around six years of bleeding if you have an average period length of five days. For some, it's less of a monthly reminder that you're not pregnant, and more of a debilitating few days of pain management. Heavy, unpredictable, long and/or painful periods can make life harder, but contraception can be really successful at managing them – in fact, it's a superpower side effect of hormonal contraception that often gets overlooked. Let's dive into two of the most common issues relating to problematic periods – heavy bleeding and pain – how to spot if these apply to you, and what can be done to manage them both with hormones and without.

## Is your period 'heavy'?

Heavy bleeding (which doctors call menorrhagia, heavy menstrual bleeding or abnormal uterine bleeding) is defined by the NHS as '80ml or more in each period, having periods that last longer than seven days, or both'.[2] Fortunately, you don't have to squeeze out your sanitary products to establish whether you have heavy periods. If you change pads or tampons every one to two hours, have to double up on period products, pass blood clots larger than 2.5 cm (about the size of a 10p coin) and bleed through your clothes or bedding a lot, these all indicate heavy bleeding and you should see your GP.

For many, there is no obvious reason for heavy bleeding. However, it can be a sign of an underlying issue, such as fibroids, pelvic inflammatory disease or endometriosis. Due to the potential range of causes, it's important to seek medical advice if you have heavy periods. A side effect of heavy bleeding can be low iron and sometimes iron-deficiency anaemia, which is when you don't have enough red blood cells to efficiently supply oxygen to your organs and muscles. Anaemia can cause symptoms like tiredness and shortness of breath – your healthcare professional can check your red blood cell and iron levels and may offer you treatment if they're low.

## Is your period pain 'normal'?

Standard period pain ('primary dysmenorrhoea' is the medical term) is caused by contractions of the uterus, which help to shed the lining each month, and the release of chemicals called prostaglandins. As with heavy bleeding, in some cases, period pain can be a symptom of an underlying condition, like fibroids or endometriosis. This is called 'secondary dysmenorrhoea'. While lots of people experience cramps in the run-up to or during their period, having pain that stops you from carrying out daily tasks is *not* normal and shouldn't be something that you put up with.

If you suffer from painful periods, notice any changes in your pain or if you get additional symptoms like pain during sex or bleeding in-between periods, speak to your doctor. When describing your pain, it's helpful for them to know: where the pain is and where it spreads to; when the pain comes on and how long it lasts; what the pain feels like; and how bad the pain is. Often a scale of pain from 0 to 10 is useful, with 0 being no pain, and 10 being the worst pain you've ever experienced. As well as what makes the pain better or worse (including sex), and any other symptoms, including with your bladder and bowels – even if you don't think they're relevant, they could be!

### Non-contraceptive treatments for heavy bleeding and period pain

Over-the-counter painkillers, like paracetamol and ibuprofen, can help with period pain. But depending on the cause of your heavy or painful periods, your doctor or pharmacist may suggest other non-hormonal treatments. These may include tranexamic acid, which stops blood clots from breaking down to reduce blood flow, or stronger non-steroidal anti-inflammatory drugs (NSAIDs) like naproxen or mefenamic acid, which can help reduce both pain and bleeding. Other things to try are placing a hot-water bottle or warm compress on the sore area. Thirty-two per cent of Lowdown users who tried this for endometriosis pain found it effective.[3] Generally, keeping warm and comfortable and doing some gentle exercises can help, but if you're looking for other treatments to try, a transcutaneous electrical nerve stimulation (TENS) machine might be an option. Nineteen per cent of our users who tried a TENS machine for endometriosis pain found it helped.[4]

Finally, some women may use progestogen tablets each month to reduce their flow, such as medroxyprogesterone (brand name Provera), but these do not act as contraceptives.

### Contraceptive treatments for heavy bleeding and period pain

Some contraceptives can make a big difference to problematic periods, while others can actually make them worse. Combined contraception (the pill, patch and ring) can make bleeds lighter and less painful. Progestogen-only methods, including the pill, implant and injection, can also help to reduce painful, heavy periods. However, irregular or prolonged bleeding (and sometimes heavier bleeding) are possible side effects, more commonly associated with progestogen-only methods, which we'll look at more closely in the next chapter. The most effective treatment for heavy periods is the hormonal coil (IUS), which releases progestogen into the uterus, thinning its lining, and which often results in periods becoming lighter, less frequent or even stopping altogether. Studies have shown in people with heavy periods the hormonal coils containing 52 mg levonorgestrel can reduce bleeding by a huge 90 per cent.[5] The copper coil can make periods heavier, longer and potentially more painful for some, so should be avoided if you already suffer from heavy bleeding.

If you're fed up with heavy or painful periods, and you use combined hormonal contraception, you can use it to stop your period altogether.

### Using contraception to skip your period

To bleed or not to bleed, that is the question. As we mentioned on page 56, 'periods' on combined hormonal contraception aren't 'real' periods, they're withdrawal bleeds, which occur

## How Lowdown users reported contraception changed their periods

Reviewers were asked: Have you noticed any changes to your periods while using this contraception? Reviewers could select more than one option.

| | Heavier periods | Lighter periods | Stopped periods |
|---|---|---|---|
| **Combined pill** | 8% | 48% | 7% |
| **Progestogen-only pill** | 5% | 8% | 45% |
| **Hormonal coil (IUS)** | 4% | 25% | 48% |
| **Implant** | 11% | 5% | 34% |
| **Copper coil (IUD)** | 69% | 3% | 3% |
| **Injection** | 5% | 5% | 70% |
| **Patch** | 8% | 37% | 6% |
| **Vaginal ring** | 0% | 50% | 6% |

| **Irregular periods** | **Spotting or breakthrough bleeding** | **No change** | **Don't know / can't tell** |
|---|---|---|---|
| 5% | 10% | 16% | 7% |
| 33% | 16% | 3% | 2% |
| 19% | 13% | 2% | 3% |
| 49% | 16% | 1% | 1% |
| 10% | 11% | 10% | 3% |
| 13% | 13% | 2% | 2% |
| 6% | 8% | 22% | 7% |
| 0% | 28% | 22% | 6% |

Analysis of The Lowdown contraception review data July 2024. 2,466 combined pill reviews, 1,298 progestogen-only pill reviews, 767 hormonal coil (IUS) reviews, 581 implant reviews, 557 copper coil (IUD) reviews, 263 injection reviews, 97 patch reviews, 18 vaginal ring reviews.

in response to the hormone-free break. This is why combined hormonal contraception can be used to stop periods altogether or to choose which months to bleed as and when suits you – e.g. making sure you don't bleed while you're on holiday. All you need to do is take it back to back without a break.

Listen closely: you do not need to have a period each month if you're using hormonal contraception. This goes for both combined and progestogen-only methods (lots of people using progestogen-only methods find their periods stop altogether). There are no specific benefits to taking the seven-day hormone-free break if you're using combined methods, either for your health or for the effectiveness of your contraception. Similarly, there's no limit to how many times you should miss your seven-day break (or skip placebo pills). So you could skip your withdrawal bleed every so often, or do it every month.

A lack of evidence-based information made lots of us believe we need to bleed each month on hormonal contraception to stay healthy. When the pill was first developed, it centred around taking a pill daily for twenty-one days followed by seven days pill-free to have a bleed that mimicked a 'real' period. We now know that this break was unnecessary; in fact, we now know there may be benefits to *not* bleeding while taking contraception. So, why was the seven-day break introduced in the first place?

One theory is that scientists and drug companies worked to create a product that attempted to mimic a 'natural' menstrual cycle to make the contraceptive pill more acceptable to influential naysayers, such as the Catholic Church. The Church saw contraception as a catalyst for loose morals and a sexual revolution (sounds appealing). Such was Catholicism's successful influence in some countries, the pill was often prescribed only to married women, and only to manage the discomfort of periods rather than as a form of contraception. There were many protests over the Church's involvement in the contraception debate, with placards and chants fuelled by the slogan: 'Keep your rosaries off my ovaries!'

Really, the guidelines advising a withdrawal bleed were mostly due to the mindset at the time the pill was developed: having monthly bleeds was seen as 'normal' and, incorrectly, necessary. It was also thought that they would serve to reassure women that their contraception was working and that they weren't pregnant. And it would allow the body a break from taking hormones, which were delivered in much higher dosages back then.[6]

The suggestion that women could safely take the pill back to back was not made public, and it's frustrating that it's only generations on that we're learning this. It's taken way too long for pill manufacturers to update their patient information, and for healthcare professionals to become familiar with 'back-to-backing' combined contraception.

Recent studies have suggested there are benefits to taking combined contraception back to back like fewer mood swings,[7] and research has argued that taking the pill continuously might even improve how effective it is.[8] When you take the pill, you're essentially putting your ovaries to sleep, interrupting your cycle to stop ovulation and prevent pregnancy. After the seven-day break your ovaries 'wake up' again, so if you forget to take your pill for a couple of days afterwards, you may ovulate and be at risk of pregnancy. Continuous pill-taking can also help alleviate the agonising symptoms of conditions like endometriosis, which we'll dive into later in this chapter.

**How to take combined contraception back-to-back**

It's like it says on the tin, just keep taking the pill every day without a break. And if you are using a combined pill that contains placebo pills, ignore them and just keep taking active pills. Some irregular bleeding and spotting are totally normal during the first few months of continuous pill taking. You might also start spotting or bleeding after running a few packets back to back. This does tend to lessen over time, though, and most women find that it becomes less of an issue when it does occur.

This rule of four could help: If you've had spotting or bleeding for more than *four* days, and it hasn't settled after twenty-one consecutive days of taking the pill, stop taking the pill for *four* days. After the four days have passed, start a new pack from the pill that matches the current day, throwing away the ones from the days you missed.

If you do decide to take a four-day or seven-day break, there's no need to use any other forms of contraception; as long as you've taken twenty-one consecutive active pills, you will continue to be protected against pregnancy.

## PMS (premenstrual syndrome) and PMDD (premenstrual dysphoric disorder)

• **PMS** is the visitor (or annoying guest you want to leave) that, for many people, rocks up each month in the days or even two weeks leading up to their period, i.e. during the luteal phase (see page 24 for a refresher). It can be the reason for a long list of physical and emotional symptoms: cramps, bloating, tender boobs, mood swings, headaches, greasy hair, dodgy sleep, appetite changes and changes to sex drive. Some people liken it to having 'period-flu'. Symptoms can vary in intensity from person to person and even between cycles, or you may be lucky and not get them at all. Because of the range in severity, and the fact that many women get mild premenstrual symptoms, the condition is unfortunately often trivialised and under-recognised by the public and health professionals. In order to confirm a diagnosis of PMS and differentiate it from other conditions, you should keep a symptom diary for two menstrual cycles in order to demonstrate the significant impact it has on day-to-day life, and that symptoms improve with your period starting.[9]

- **Premenstrual dysphoric disorder (PMDD)** is a severe form of PMS, with diagnostic criteria from the American Psychiatric Association focused on mood and psychiatric symptoms.[10] A large study of 50,000 women determined at least 1.6 per cent of us experience it, and many think this is an underestimate, quoting more like one in twenty.[11] PMDD symptoms are next-level in terms of extremity. In one survey, around three-quarters of people with PMDD had suicidal thoughts and over one-third had attempted suicide.[12] For some, this may also include exacerbation of an underlying mental health problem. It's extraordinary to think that a large number of people are battling these symptoms for a large part of each month.

We still don't fully understand the causes behind PMS and PMDD but it's thought to be down to hormonal fluctuations over the month, and sensitivity to changes in brain chemistry as oestrogen and the chemical serotonin drop in the luteal phase of the cycle leading up to bleeding. Like so many other aspects of women's health, more funding for research is desperately needed to understand the cause and to find better treatment options.

## How is PMDD diagnosed?

To be diagnosed with PMDD, you need to have at least five out of eleven defined symptoms, including one related to your mood (such as mood swings and/or feelings of sadness or anxiety). They must be present in the final week before your period and cause significant distress or interfere with work, school or usual activities. They must start to *improve* with the start of your period, and become *minimal* or absent in the week after your period.[13]

Symptoms include: mood swings or crying, lasting irritability or anger, feelings of sadness or despair, tension or anxiety, lack of interest in activities and relationships, trouble concentrating and muddled thinking, tiredness or low energy, food cravings or binge eating, trouble sleeping, feeling out of control, physical symptoms like cramps, breast tenderness, bloating, or muscle or joint pain.[14]

PMDD may not be diagnosed or be misdiagnosed for many reasons, one being that symptoms can cross over with other conditions like depression and anxiety. Seek support from your GP early, especially as symptoms are distressing and impact on your life. Keep a diary of your symptoms (even if you're not sure which ones are related to PMDD) and track them for at least two cycles. Record any interventions that help your symptoms, too. There are free and paid-for apps that can make this easier, or keep track via pen and paper or on your phone. This will be crucial for your GP to help with a diagnosis. And please remember that if you do feel very low or even suicidal, help is just a phone call away; please see page 359 for available services.

## Contraceptive treatments for PMS and PMDD

For some, hormonal contraception is a really effective way of keeping PMS symptoms in check. Research has found that newer types of combined contraceptive pills containing oestrogen and the newer progestogen drospirenone (such as Yasmin, Lucette, Drovelis and Eloine) can improve PMS and

PMDD symptoms, especially when taken back to back.[15] This is because it prevents the usual hormonal fluctuations over the course of the menstrual cycle that can trigger the symptoms.

Unfortunately, some people find taking hormonal contraception makes them feel even worse. Everyone is different and our sensitivity to hormonal changes, as well as the unique balance of hormones in our bodies, means that we all react differently. The culprit is usually synthetic progestins, which some women are really sensitive to and can cause PMS-like side effects such as mood changes, bloating and sore boobs. Progestogen-only contraception alone is not therefore usually recommended for those with PMS, but the data to support this is lacking and the hormonal coils or the progestin drospirenone may be better tolerated.[16]

### Non-contraceptive treatments for PMS and PMDD

- **Lifestyle** As with most things, boosting sleep, eating well, exercising and limiting alcohol and caffeine is never going to be a bad thing. But if you're feeling overloaded in the days leading up to your period, there's no harm in going to bed early with an episode or two of trashy TV that requires zero brain power to help you de-stress.
- **Pain relief** Over-the-counter medication such as paracetamol or ibuprofen can help with cramps, and joint or muscle pain.
- **Cognitive behavioural therapy (CBT)** This can be particularly useful for anyone who suffers from chronic illness and should be offered to anyone with severe PMS.[17] CBT is a type of talking therapy which can help you process the emotional and psychological aspects of what you're going through. Your GP can help you access this through the NHS (see the Resources section), or it can be paid for privately.

- **Supplements** There isn't yet enough research to bring advice on supplements into clinical recommendation. However, there is some evidence to suggest that calcium and vitamin D, vitamin B6, magnesium, isoflavones, St John's wort and agnus castus (though, not recommended if you're trying to conceive or are breastfeeding) may reduce PMS symptoms.[18] Always speak to a healthcare professional (usually a pharmacist) before taking any supplements, particularly if you're already taking any other type of medication or remedies.
- **Complementary therapies** Unfortunately, there hasn't been enough research into the impact of therapies such as acupuncture and reflexology for treating PMS but anecdotally, some people find it helps them.
- **Antidepressants** The most common type of antidepressants are called selective serotonin reuptake inhibitors (SSRIs), which have been shown to be effective for PMS and PMDD.[19] These include tablets like fluoxetine, sertraline, escitalopram or citalopram. For severe PMS or PMDD, these tablets can be taken for half your cycle, in a two week on, two week off fashion, or continuously, i.e. every day. Taking these during your luteal phase before your period can really help symptoms (not just psychological symptoms: there's evidence physical symptoms can improve too) and doesn't appear to cause any antidepressant withdrawal symptoms.[20]
- **Gonadotropin releasing hormone (GnRH) analogues** These typically come as injections and work by inducing temporary menopause, and so can relieve symptoms of severe PMS and PMDD for some people.[21] It tends to be considered a last-resort treatment because it brings with it potential side effects such as loss of bone density (causing bones to become weak and more at risk of breaks) and menopausal symptoms. It should be combined with hormone replacement therapy (see next point), which reduces bone density loss.

- **Hormone replacement therapy (HRT)** HRT is sometimes prescribed to treat PMS and PMDD when other options haven't worked or are not suitable (usually in the form of oestrogen patches and either tablet progesterone for two weeks a month or the hormonal coil). It works by overriding your cycle with continuous daily oestrogen, so that you don't have periods. However, it's important to note that for some women, especially those who are sensitive to synthetic progestogens, the hormonal coil can make PMS/PMDD symptoms worse initially, and the tablet progesterone can also have its own side effects.
- **Hysterectomy and oophorectomy** This is a surgical procedure which permanently removes the uterus and ovaries. This means the menstrual cycle stops for ever and, hopefully, so too do PMS and PMDD symptoms. This is a radical treatment option that requires very serious consideration to weigh up the pros and cons. It means there will be no chance of pregnancy and hormone replacement therapy is required to manage menopausal symptoms as you don't want to swap one set of symptoms for another. In reality, this is rarely performed for PMS as usually people will respond to alternative less extreme treatments.

## Menstrual migraine

Many people get headaches around the time of their period and for some these can be in the form of migraine attacks. The main trigger for menstrual migraines is thought to be the drop in oestrogen levels that occurs just before your period, similar to PMS. There is no test to diagnose menstrual migraines, but keeping a symptom diary can, once again, help you recognise a pattern. As well as the usual migraine treatments that focus on pain and symptom relief, contraception can help. Options are either to take the combined pill continuously without a break to avoid the drop in oestrogen or, for those with migraine with aura (more on this in Chapter 6), progestogen-only methods can also work well. However, headaches can also be a side effect of hormonal contraception for some people (see Chapter 5) and irregular bleeding associated with progestogen-only methods can be accompanied by migraine.[22] For more info about lifestyle changes and treatments for migraine, and for tips about how to distinguish between a headache and a migraine, see The Migraine Trust (details in Resources).

## Acne

A whopping 95 per cent of us are affected by acne at some point in our lives, with 20–35 per cent of people having moderate to severe acne. It's characterised by blockage of the pores in the skin causing spots, affecting the face 99 per cent of the time, but also the chest or back.[23] Several processes contribute to the formation of acne, but when it comes to contraception, it's the androgens we'll focus on.

Our skin glands are really sensitive to androgens (flip back to page 42 for a refresher on these). Androgens cause glands in your skin to produce excess amounts of oil (called sebum) and also thicken hair follicles, causing blocked pores. Excess sebum interacts with usually harmless bacteria on the skin, which then causes spots. This is why acne is a common symptom of PCOS, because the ovaries produce more androgens. Oestrogen, one of the main hormones involved in the menstrual cycle, has the opposite effect on sebum production. Experts think oestrogen reduces sebum by negative feedback on the ovaries to reduce androgen production – which is why you might be more spotty at certain points in your cycle.

Combined hormonal contraception is a recommended

treatment for acne. Studies show that women with acne who take the combined pill tend to see an improvement in the number of spots and the severity of their acne compared to those who aren't on hormonal contraception.[24] Because of this, some people are prescribed certain pill brands to clear their skin even if they don't actually need contraception. There's not much research on which brand is best, but one study found pills containing the progestogen drospirenone are the most helpful for preventing acne. It also concluded that pills containing levonorgestrel and norethisterone (also called norethindrone) were the least helpful.[25] See our pill groups table in Chapter 2 for a breakdown of pill ingredients.

## Polycystic ovary syndrome (PCOS)

Despite the name (which would be better suited to something like 'Paused Egg Syndrome'), PCOS doesn't actually involve cysts on the ovaries. Rather, the ovaries are enlarged, with multiple follicles, which are fluid-filled sacs, containing eggs. The cause of PCOS isn't fully understood, but it centres around a hormonal imbalance in the body, with the over-production of androgens and a reduced sensitivity to insulin, the hormone which regulates blood sugar levels. People with PCOS are often somewhat resistant to the effects of insulin, which then leads to higher-than-normal levels of insulin in the blood, which causes the ovaries to produce too much testosterone.

PCOS affects the function of the ovaries and is experienced by around 10 per cent of women and people who have ovaries.[26] The main symptom is irregular, less frequent periods due to irregular ovulation or sometimes not ovulating at all. Other common symptoms of PCOS include weight gain, excessive hair growth on the face and body (hirsutism), hair loss, acne and difficulty getting pregnant (irregular less frequent periods = less frequent ovulation and fewer fertile days, but pregnancy can often be achieved naturally or with medical help).[27] At The Lowdown we often hear from people with PCOS who have other symptoms, such as bloating, fatigue and even snoring. However, everyone is different, so some people experience more symptoms than others.

PCOS also affects women of colour differently than white women – something which is not yet fully understood but may be because of a predisposition of some ethnicities to cardiovascular disease and diabetes. Health inequity in the UK, and much of the world, is rife. There desperately needs to be more research carried out into how certain gynaecological conditions affect people of colour, and better pathways for care that help marginalised groups get diagnosed with conditions like PCOS in the first place.

**PCOS explained**

Professor Colin Duncan is a Principal Investigator in the Centre for Reproductive Health at the University of Edinburgh. He runs a research laboratory that studies polycystic ovary syndrome. We asked him where we are currently with understanding what causes PCOS . . .

'PCOS runs in families and is more commonly shared by identical twins rather than non-identical twins. That means there is likely to be a genetic component. However, all the research has only found genetic markers that account for a small fraction of PCOS. It is likely that it's a combination of genetic and environmental factors, and that the environment that is present before birth has a role in programming later

PCOS. Nonetheless, we do not fully understand the causes. Our research has shown that exposure to some extra male type hormones like testosterone before birth seems to have a role to play. We have given pregnant sheep a bit of extra male type hormone during the middle of pregnancy, and studied their offspring who develop the features of PCOS, such as weight gain and irregular ovulation. We are now using our discoveries about why weight gain is more likely to occur to try to help those with PCOS.'

### How is PCOS diagnosed?

It's not always possible to diagnose PCOS based on symptoms alone, but if you have two or more of the following symptoms, you may have polycystic ovary syndrome (if other potential causes have been ruled out):[28]

- Irregular periods (i.e. if the gap between them is less than twenty-one days or more than thirty-five days in adult premenopausal women) or no periods.
- High levels of androgens. These can be detected in blood tests or your healthcare professional can look for clinical signs of high androgens, such as acne, excessive hair growth on the face or body or female pattern hair loss.
- Ultrasound scans showing you have the appearance of polycystic ovaries – which aren't actually cysts but follicles, remember. There is a list of criteria to tick off which classify your ovaries as having 'PCOS morphology' OR a raised blood level of a hormone called anti-müllerian hormone (AMH). AMH may be used in place of an ultrasound. AMH levels have been used in fertility

> clinics for years and high levels have recently been shown to closely relate to how the ovaries look on ultrasound. However, it is likely to take some time before AMH blood testing is regularly used in clinical practice.

It's important to know that an ultrasound and AMH testing can't be used to formally diagnose PCOS within eight years of you starting your periods, as many women will still naturally have lots of follicles on their ovaries.[29] It's also interesting that women can have PCOS *without* having the classical signs on an ultrasound scan. And women can have polycystic-looking ovaries on a scan but without having any of the symptoms to classify as having the full syndrome. Sounds complicated, doesn't it? It reflects the fact that PCOS is a syndrome – a recognised pattern of symptoms – rather than a condition with a single cause or definitive test and why researchers suspect that classification and diagnosis of PCOS may change in the upcoming years.

## Contraceptive options to help manage PCOS

There is currently no cure for PCOS but the symptoms can be improved and managed. The best type of contraception for PCOS varies from person to person, so it's a good idea to speak to a healthcare professional with an interest in gynaecology or sexual and reproductive health to guide you through the options. One way of managing the symptoms of PCOS is by using hormonal contraception, like the combined contraceptive pill, the patch or the vaginal ring. These help regulate the menstrual cycle and reduce the level of androgens in the body. Combined pills that contain anti-androgenic progestogens (such as Yasmin, Lucette, Drovelis or Eloine) can be a good choice for managing the androgenic symptoms of PCOS. But many women find the brands containing

**PCOS**

Symptoms 8–10 years   30 years old

**PCOS experience**

I'm thirty and I was diagnosed with PCOS in 2020 after suspecting I had the condition for a long time. I requested a blood test, and this was enough, with my other symptoms, for the GP to confirm I had high testosterone levels, and to give a PCOS diagnosis. From my teenage years, I have always had irregular periods, ranging from two- to six-week cycles (which were often heavy), fatigue, suffered on and off with acne and when I started suffering with hirsutism I knew something really wasn't right. Post diagnosis and taking myself off the pill to see how my body was without synthetic hormones, my symptoms went from a bit out of control post pill, to becoming more manageable with diet and lifestyle changes. Now, three years on, I feel like my efforts have plateaued and I'm struggling with extreme fatigue, bad skin, hair, weight gain and anxiety. My periods range from thirty to fifty days in length and are, yet again, becoming very heavy and painful. No doctor so far has been able to help me, other than to suggest I go back on the pill. The pill masks symptoms therefore never gets to the root cause, which was the reason I took myself off them in the first place.

Shared on **thelowdown.com**

androgenic progestogens work well too, due to their oestrogen content. Dianette is a combined pill brand containing an anti-androgenic progestogen called cyproterone acetate. However, it's only licensed to be used for severe acne and hirsutism (which can be caused by PCOS), and although it provides effective contraception in those who use it, it should not be used just for contraception.[30] Women with PCOS who don't have regular bleeds (at least one every three months, i.e. four per year) are at increased risk of having a thickened uterus lining (doctors call the uterus lining the endometrium). This can increase the risk of cancer of the uterus, so it's important to either trigger a bleed every three months *or* keep the uterus lining thin. Combined contraception keeps the uterus lining thin, as do all of the progestogen-only contraceptives (the hormonal coil, implant, injection or progestogen-only pill). Many people will also prefer the benefit of no or fewer periods associated with hormonal contraception.

If you're not using hormonal contraception to keep the uterus lining thin, and don't have at least four periods a year, progestin tablets called medroxyprogesterone (that are not used as contraception) should be used for ten to fourteen days every three months to trigger bleeds and protect against endometrial (uterus) cancer.

### Non-contraceptive options to help manage PCOS

If you have PCOS, the same health and well-being guidelines that help with everyday life apply: eating a nutrient-rich, varied diet; exercising (but not to excess); reducing caffeine; limiting alcohol; lowering stress and enjoying quality sleep. Aiming for a healthy weight is also beneficial – which is often extra tricky for those with PCOS as the condition can make it easier to gain weight and more difficult to lose it.[31] Similarly, if you're feeling tired, stressed and worn down with PCOS, it can be even harder to feel motivated. Cooking a nutritious meal at the end of a long day or rolling out the exercise mat may understandably be the last thing you feel like doing. There is no evidence that a particular diet or exercise is better for weight loss if you have PCOS, rather the 'best' one is the one that works for *you*, that you'll feel able to stick with. Let go of the idea of restriction and punishment and think about including foods and movement that nourish you. From The Lowdown data, 31 per cent of people with PCOS told us exercise was effective or very effective at managing their PCOS symptoms; 28 per cent said the same for dietary changes and 17 per cent for stress management.[32]

- **Inositol** Inositol is a naturally occurring sugar found in supplements which can help treat the symptoms of PCOS. The supplements are readily available to buy and can be taken by most women. It may improve cycle regularity and reduce testosterone, glucose and body mass index (BMI) for some women but the evidence is limited.[33]
- **Metformin** This drug, which is typically used for type 2 diabetes, can improve the body's sensitivity to insulin. In the UK, doctors can prescribe this for PCOS as it may help with weight loss, insulin sensitivity and can help induce ovulation.
- **Spironolactone** Drospirenone, an anti-androgenic progestogen, is derived from spironolactone. This drug is used to treat cardiovascular conditions, such as heart failure or high blood pressure, but can sometimes be used by specialists off licence to treat acne and hirsutism associated with PCOS if traditional acne treatments or hair removal options haven't worked. Drospirenone, an anti-androgenic progestin, is derived from spironolactone.

---

**Q:** I am currently taking hormonal contraception to manage PCOS but would like to start trying for a baby. Will stopping the pill lead my symptoms to worsen? Is there anything else I can do that won't impact my fertility?

**A:** As the combined pill is an effective treatment for PCOS, unfortunately stopping it might make your symptoms worsen. However, if you're stopping to try to conceive, this is an ideal opportunity to really concentrate on the lifestyle changes that can improve PCOS, as they are likely to help your fertility and support a healthy pregnancy too. Try to stop smoking and drinking alcohol and start taking vitamin D and folic acid (ask your pharmacist or GP for the correct dose for you). Inositol supplements can help regulate your cycle and alleviate PCOS symptoms and are safe to take if you fall pregnant.[34]

## Fibroids

Fibroids, fibroids, so common but often forgotten! So common, in fact, that 70 per cent of white women and 80 per cent of Black women will have a fibroid during their lifetime, with 30 per cent suffering from severe symptoms.[35] Despite this, there is little awareness and research about one of the most common women's health conditions.

### What are fibroids?

Fibroids are non-cancerous growths that develop in or on the uterus, made up of muscle and tissue. They can vary in size and number and diagnosis is usually confirmed with imaging, often an ultrasound scan. Fibroids are classified based on their location: within the uterine wall, inside the uterus, on the outer surface of the uterus or attached by a stalk. Many women with fibroids have no symptoms, and only find out once they have an ultrasound scan. Others may experience heavy or longer periods, pelvic, leg or back pain, constipation or the need to pass urine more often. In some cases, large fibroids can distend the abdomen and make someone look pregnant when they're not. The exact cause of fibroids is unknown, but factors like genetics and hormonal changes may contribute.

### How to treat fibroids

Treatment options range from medications to manage symptoms, including hormonal contraceptives, to more invasive interventional or surgical procedures, depending on the individual and severity of symptoms. Inserting a coil can be more challenging with large fibroids, especially if they are large enough to change the size and shape of the uterus, and the risk of the coil falling out may be higher. In these cases coil fitting should be done by a specialist.[36] Sometimes the coil may not be suitable at all if it can't be sited correctly.

## Endometriosis

Endometriosis is another common health condition that affects one in ten women of child-bearing age[37] – that's 190 million people globally: almost the population of Brazil. It has always been described as a disease of the reproductive system; however, research now suggests that it's a whole-body inflammatory condition where endometrial-like cells, similar to the ones in the lining of the uterus, are found in other parts of the body, such as on the ovaries, bladder, bowels, pelvic and abdominal walls. In rare cases, they can even be found further afield like the lining of the lungs. These cells react to the ebb and flow of hormones during the menstrual cycle and each month they thicken and then shed like your uterus lining. But unlike menstrual blood, there is no way for bleeding from endometrial deposits outside the uterus to leave the body, and this is what causes inflammation, pain and scar tissue (also known as adhesions).

Like PCOS, people with endometriosis experience a range of symptoms in different severities. For some, it won't have much impact on everyday life (sometimes people have the condition without even being aware of it), whereas for others it may be all-consuming. Chronic pain (often around the pelvis, tummy, back and legs), exhaustion and difficulty conceiving are common symptoms, which in turn may have a knock-on effect on a person's ability to work, enjoy hobbies and socialise. This in turn can understandably affect other aspects of well-being, including mental health, sometimes leading to depression. We know from The Lowdown's review data that 83 per cent of those with endometriosis who shared their experience on our website reported symptoms of depression and/or anxiety and 92 per cent reported tiredness or fatigue.[38]

### Symptoms of endometriosis[39]

- Painful periods which may start from one to two days before bleeding and continue through your period.
- Heavy periods, long periods, spotting in-between periods or losing old, dark blood before your period starts.
- Pelvic, back or leg pain.
- Deep pain within your pelvis or abdomen during sex or internal medical examinations.
- Pain or bleeding going to the toilet (when passing urine or opening the bowels), especially while on your period.
- Difficulty getting pregnant (though the majority of endometriosis suffers do get pregnant naturally, more on page 273).
- Fatigue, lethargy and mood changes (hardly a surprise given the symptoms above!).

**Endometriosis**
Symptoms 5–8 years 36 years old

**Endometriosis experience**

I started my periods aged ten and was having a week off school every month due to pain. I was given the contraceptive pill aged eleven, which gave me my life back. My period pain returned aged twenty-eight and I knew straightaway something was wrong. I had painful/heavy periods, painful ovulation and sex also became painful. When they found endometriosis on my first laparoscopy, I felt relieved there was finally an answer. I had two laparoscopies to remove endometriosis. I always get short-term relief, but my symptoms return. My symptoms are currently the worst they've ever been and now involve bladder and bowel pain. I'm constantly fatigued and need to take time off work to rest. My latest MRI showed adenomyosis, an endometrial ovarian cyst and an ovary stuck to my bowel. It's important to know that endometriosis rarely shows on scans so don't take negative findings as proof you don't have it. Living with my symptoms is hard. This is made worse by NHS wait times which mean getting help takes a long time. We know our bodies the best and if you suspect endometriosis, keep pushing for answers. Painful periods are not normal and we shouldn't be left in debilitating pain.

Shared on **thelowdown.com**

## How to get a diagnosis

If your day-to-day quality of life is affected by the symptoms of endometriosis (or any medical condition), it's important to see a healthcare professional. When The Lowdown's doctors speak to people with suspected or diagnosed endometriosis, they often describe their symptoms as 'debilitating'.

Frustratingly, the cause of endometriosis isn't yet fully understood and, disappointingly, the average time it takes for a woman in the UK to receive a definitive diagnosis is nearly nine years from when symptoms begin.[40] Often it's not a straightforward journey and you are likely to see a lot of healthcare professionals during this time. So, symptom control (coming up) is important to keep on top of it while you pursue a diagnosis. Given around 10 per cent of women in their reproductive years suffer from endometriosis, this is a staggering number of people whose everyday life is affected.

There is currently no definitive *simple* test or scan that determines whether or not someone has endometriosis. Symptoms are variable for each person and can overlap with other problems such as irritable bowel syndrome (IBS), polycystic ovary syndrome or sexually transmitted infections, meaning it can sometimes be difficult to pinpoint as endometriosis. The first step is to speak to your GP about your symptoms (keeping a diary or writing down a list and taking it to your appointment can be helpful). They will examine you and arrange for an ultrasound scan of your pelvis if they suspect endometriosis. However, an ultrasound won't always pick up endometriosis, especially if the deposits are spread across the pelvis, or if the scan isn't performed by a specialist.[41] This means that you can't rule out a diagnosis based on a normal ultrasound scan and if your symptoms are still suggestive of endometriosis, referral to a gynaecologist and further investigation is needed.[42]

The current most effective way of diagnosing endometriosis is via a laparoscopy, which is a keyhole operation, under general anaesthetic, whereby a camera is inserted into the abdomen and pelvis through small cuts in the tummy to look for endometrial deposits. If found, deposits may be treated at the same time, by being cut or burned away and any scar tissue that has formed can be removed. Not everyone needs a laparoscopy for diagnosis or wants one, especially if treatment is helpful. As with any surgery, there are potential risks that your doctor will discuss with you before you make a choice.

For those who embark on the surgical option, hormonal contraception is often recommended to prevent endometriosis symptoms returning after surgical treatment.[43] You may choose to start hormonal contraception as a way to relieve your symptoms before a diagnosis is formally made. If you choose to wait for diagnosis via laparoscopy, specialists recommend starting hormonal contraception as soon as possible after surgery. Options such as the hormonal coil (IUS) can even be inserted at the time of your surgery while you are under anaesthetic.

Whatever your course of action, getting a diagnosis can feel life changing for some and hugely validating for those who have spent years seeking help, advocating for themselves and being on waiting lists for specialist care.

**Alice's experience with endometriosis and diagnosis**

Alice, The Lowdown's founder and CEO, was diagnosed with endometriosis when she was twenty-six. Here she shares her experience of being diagnosed:

'Like most women, it took me years to be diagnosed.

I had always suffered from rather dramatic period pains, but in my early twenties I started to find sex eye-wateringly uncomfortable. It was only after convincing the 100th doctor that I didn't have an STI, and insisting on having an internal ultrasound, that I was able to get referred to see a gynaecologist to get these symptoms properly investigated.

'I had my first laparoscopy surgery in 2015 and remember waking up from the anaesthetic and feeling so relieved when the doctor told me they'd found endometriosis deposits around my uterus. Although it was tough news, it felt so vindicating to finally have a reason, and a cause for this unexplained pain.

'I found the recovery from laparoscopic surgery slower than I expected. While it's keyhole surgery and I've been left with some tiny scars on my stomach, the effects of the anaesthetic and pain relief meant it took me a fair few weeks to get back to "normal". But the procedure did help alleviate my pain, and during the surgery they fitted me with a hormonal coil (IUS), which was the best contraceptive method I've tried – it stopped my periods and cramping pains for many years.

'We desperately need less invasive, quicker ways to be diagnosed with endometriosis and more treatment options. The waiting lists for surgery like this are too long, and costs too high, and this puts living pain-free on hold for millions of women worldwide.'

### Treatment and management

You might be surprised to hear that for some people (one study quotes 13 per cent[44]), endometriosis can get better of its own accord without any treatment – though doctors don't always know why, the mysterious condition that it is. However, as the symptoms can impact on your quality of life so much, the majority of people opt for treatment – with the right support, symptoms can be managed.

You might have heard a myth that getting pregnant can cure endometriosis but there's no evidence to support this, despite an Australian study finding that women were actually being told this.[45] While being pregnant may temporarily ease symptoms, it's not a magical cure. In fact, endometriosis can make it harder to get pregnant in the first place, which we go into in Chapter 9.

### Hormonal contraception as treatment for endometriosis

Hormonal contraceptives can be a game changer for those suffering from endometriosis. Combined hormonal contraceptives stop ovulation and thin the uterus lining. This means that endometrial deposits can become smaller without the hormonal stimulation of the menstrual cycle. Taking the combined pill back to back could offer the greatest relief by minimising the number of bleeds you have. The 52 mg levonorgestrel hormonal coil (IUS), like the Mirena, is also a popular choice. Typically, it can make periods lighter and one study showed that after five years 42 per cent of people who used it had no bleeding at all and nearly 90 per cent had no periods or only spotting or light bleeding.[46] The progestogen-only pill, implant and injection can also help symptoms but aren't considered 'first-line treatment' because there has been less research into these methods. Medroxyprogesterone is a hormonal treatment that doesn't act as a contraceptive and there are also specialist medications and injections that can be used to stop your cycle to help symptoms.

## Effectiveness of treatments for endometriosis

| Treatment | % of all reviewers who tried this treatment | % of those reviewers who reported it as 'effective' or 'very effective' |
|---|---|---|
| *Lifestyle* | | |
| Dietary changes | 62% | 23% |
| Stress management | 61% | 23% |
| Exercise | 78% | 15% |
| *Medication* | | |
| Codeine | 54% | 42% |
| Tramadol | 22% | 49% |
| Naproxen | 43% | 24% |
| Ibuprofen | 85% | 12% |
| Tranexamic acid | 34% | 28% |
| Mefenamic acid | 41% | 23% |
| Antidepressants | 27% | 23% |
| Progestogens | 20% | 22% |
| GnRH analogues | 8% | 31% |
| Voltarol | 38% | 7% |
| Diclofenac | 13% | 10% |
| Danazol | 6% | 11% |
| *Treatments* | | |
| Pelvic health physiotherapy | 13% | 43% |
| Acupuncture | 13% | 30% |
| Massage | 26% | 12% |
| Osteopathy | 5% | 25% |

Analysis of The Lowdown endometriosis experience data July 2024
(156 endometriosis experiences)

### Non-hormonal treatments for endometriosis

As per the suggestions for those suffering with PCOS, do what you can to look after yourself in other ways: focusing on diet, exercise and sleep and reducing alcohol can help you feel better day to day.

- **Painkillers** like good old paracetamol and ibuprofen, or stronger prescription medications may be needed for those really bad days. Your doctor can help advise which pain medications are suitable, balancing the side effects and risks.
- **Pelvic physiotherapy** is a really underutilised treatment that can work wonders for endometriosis by focusing on exercises to relieve tension and pain. Ask your GP for a referral.
- **Complementary therapies,** especially acupuncture, are increasingly being researched as a treatment option for pelvic pain and painful periods[47] – hallmark symptoms of endometriosis, with some evidence of benefit.

## Adenomyosis

Adenomyosis is NOT endometriosis, as people may commonly think. It is a condition where the tissue that normally lines the inside of the uterus (endometrium) grows into the muscular wall of the uterus (myometrium), as opposed to endometriosis, where tissue similar to the endometrium is found *outside* the uterus. Like in endometriosis, this tissue thickens and bleeds with the menstrual cycle each month, causing the uterine walls to thicken and enlarge, often causing heavy, painful periods and pelvic pain. Some women with adenomyosis may also experience pain during sex and chronic pelvic pain. We don't know exactly what causes it and although it seems to be more common in women in their forties who have had children, this might be because the symptoms are different and it's less well recognised in the early stages and at a younger age.[48] Adenomyosis may be diagnosed on an ultrasound scan or by an MRI. Treatment options include medications to manage symptoms, especially hormonal contraceptives, with the 52 mg levonorgestrel hormonal coils recommended as first line treatment.[49] Surgical procedures including hysterectomy are also an option.

## What is the future for these conditions?

Our Lowdown research lead and super-intelligent clinical researcher Dr Becky Mawson always keeps us up to date with the latest in women's health advances. And here is her take on the future of conditions like PCOS and endo . . .

'The future management of many of these conditions will likely change dramatically over the next decade as we research more about them. Due to a lack of funding for women's health research, many conditions are still misunderstood. Treatment is often a mix of guesswork and trial and error. As we understand more about what causes some people to be affected by conditions like endometriosis and PCOS, we can look at better ways to prevent them rather than treat the symptoms.

'Many are calling for PCOS to be renamed as it focuses on issues with ovaries, when actually, the issue is more complex about the way the pituitary gland in the brain works as well as our metabolism. Women can have normal-looking ovaries with a diagnosis of PCOS, which causes great confusion. It is likely that different types of conditions have been put under the umbrella of PCOS and as we understand more about causes, we can start to tailor management to more precision treatments. For those with symptoms which are more related to weight gain and insulin resistance, it is likely treatments will focus on how sugar is used by the body and use diabetes treatments. Studies are underway at the moment looking at the use of metformin (diabetes medication) compared to semaglutide (Ozempic injection) for managing PCOS.[50] For those with symptoms of high levels of androgens but no issues with weight, there may be different causes which we probably miss at present because we don't look for them.[51] This may include the pituitary gland in the brain or the adrenal gland in the kidney, which produces high levels of the androgen hormones. More targeted treatments in the future may help reduce these levels without impacting fertility; drugs like spironolactone, for example, might give researchers options for management.

'Endometriosis is a condition that is poorly understood and has a long delay in diagnosis. We don't understand how it changes over time either; for example, does someone who is treated with hormones in their earlier years have less endometriosis than those who haven't been treated? There is a race in the research world to design a reliable way of diagnosing and monitoring endometriosis, some looking at markers in blood, saliva, poo and even menstrual blood. There is also a move towards trying to diagnose endometriosis by either an advanced ultrasound scan or an MRI scan, which would avoid keyhole surgery, which is often used now. The dream is that anyone with suspected endometriosis would have an advanced ultrasound by an endometriosis specialist, and they would be able to map where the problems are. That way, surgery would be targeted to exactly where the endometriosis was, and the surgeon would have an idea of how major the operation would be. There is some exciting work being done at the moment looking at gut bacteria and endometriosis; the scientists are looking at whether treating the gut bacteria might help cure endometriosis.[52]

'With all these reproductive health conditions, the first step is to understand the cause, and then scientists can look for a cure or treatment. There are a lot of exciting advances happening at the moment, but reproductive health still receives only a very small amount of public funding. We need to push for equal funding for reproductive health conditions as compared to things like cancer, heart disease and infection.'

## Sexually transmitted infections (STIs)

There are many different types of STIs. They are all passed on through sexual contact, meaning if you've had vaginal, oral or anal sex, or even shared sex toys with someone who has an STI, you could contract one – or several. The most common infections are chlamydia, gonorrhoea, herpes, genital warts, syphilis, trichomoniasis and finally human immunodeficiency virus (HIV). There are helpful resources on The Lowdown's website on each of these, as well as from the NHS or World Health Organization (WHO). Anyone can catch an STI, whether you've had one partner or one hundred, and STIs like chlamydia and gonorrhoea can be contracted more than once.

Symptoms of an STI vary according to the infection, but common ones might include pain when peeing, unusual discharge, abdominal pain, rash, warts, flu-like symptoms and bleeding after sex. However, many STIs are asymptomatic, meaning you could happily be going about your daily life with no telltale signs of infection, which is why taking precautions and regular screening are essential. Different infections require different treatments, but often, antibiotics are prescribed.

---

**Q:** You can only catch an STI through penetrative sex, right?

**A:** Nope. An STI can be passed on in semen, pre-cum and vaginal fluids (so sex toys should be washed thoroughly after each use). Some STIs, such as genital herpes, can be passed on through skin-to-skin contact. HIV and hepatitis B and C can also be passed on when blood is exchanged.

---

## Taking action

Safe sex is everyone's responsibility, so be prepared yourself by having condoms and testing regularly. If you're not in the habit of testing regularly, and you're sexually active, try to reframe your thinking around it. Incorporate it into your well-being routine, just like going to the dentist, optician or for cervical screening tests.

- **Prevention** Using condoms the moment sexual contact occurs is the most effective way to prevent getting an STI, but they do not guarantee that you won't get an STI. Male condoms are considered more effective at preventing the spread of STIs (as well as pregnancy) than female condoms as they are generally easier to use more effectively. If you've used a condom and it splits, you are at risk of getting an STI (and/or potentially becoming pregnant), so you'll need to get tested.
- **Testing** For anyone who is sexually active but not in a long term monogamous relationship, an STI and HIV test at least every twelve months is recommended, or any time you change sexual partner.[53] This is particularly important for diagnosis of infections that do not show any immediate symptoms, meaning you could quite easily have an STI without knowing it, and potentially pass it on to a partner (who in turn may unknowingly pass it on to someone else, and on and on it may go). If you've never tested before, the thought of having an STI can be daunting, thanks to societal stigma. But trust us, it's easier to get tested and treated than avoid it and hope for the best.

If you think you might have been exposed to an STI or if

you have changed sexual partners (or might be about to), your local sexual health clinic will organise free testing for you. If you don't have any symptoms or don't require an examination you may be able to do your own vaginal swabs (men are usually asked to provide a urine sample). You'll also usually be offered blood tests as part of STI screening. If you have a suspected infection, a healthcare professional will usually examine you and take a swab of the affected area. At-home self-testing kits are available (for free in the UK), whereby you take a blood or urine sample, or a swab, and post it off for testing, after which results will be texted or emailed to you, generally a few days later. Anyone with symptoms should get seen in person. Your local sexual health clinic are the experts in how to spot STI symptoms, when's best to test, and everything else you might need to know about STIs. To find your local sexual health clinic, head to the link in Resources.

- **Talking about STIs** Many people feel embarrassed or to blame when they get an STI, especially when it's 'for life', like herpes or HIV. The best way to destigmatise STIs is to talk about them more openly and reframe them from something life-changing, dirty and rare to what they really are – super common and easily treatable, especially when treatment is prompt. It's also totally possible to live a normal life with HIV or herpes without transmitting it to anyone else.

We wouldn't feel embarrassed to tell someone we'd caught any other type of virus, like a cold, so let's open the lid on STI chat. The problem with feeling shame over STIs is that it can prevent us from taking action. The best way to make sure you don't pass anything on is to know what symptoms to look for, ask your partners their status, and talk about your own, whether it's positive or negative.

- **How to tell someone you have an STI** Telling someone you have an STI should be less of a confession of guilt or shame, and more like a helpful disclosure of facts. It's of course really important to tell someone that you have an STI due to possible health risks for all involved, but the reason so many people find it hard to disclose is due to fear of backlash and rejection. When it comes to discussing your status with a partner, you could try . . .

- 'This is hard for me to talk about, but I wanted to let you know I recently tested positive for [STI]. I'd love to have an open, non-judgemental conversation about this, and decide what to do next.'
- 'Hey, I've been noticing [symptoms] and I wanted to let you know I think I have [STI], so I'm going to get tested. We should do this together as you might need to test, too.'
- 'Before we take things further, I want to let you know that I have herpes. I haven't had an outbreak in [an amount of time], and there's a low chance of you getting it. If you want to ask me any more questions about this, I'm happy to chat about it. I hope you appreciate my honesty.'

If you feel you can't speak to your partner directly, your sexual health clinic will help you do this confidentially.

# 5

# Side effects explained

A number of side effects are reported by people taking contraception, from emotional changes affecting mood and sex drive to physical ones such as bleeding, acne and weight gain. While research has confirmed a link between hormonal contraception and some of these symptoms, frustratingly, many other side effects are still considered 'anecdotal'. There is still limited research into the many reported side effects of hormonal contraception and how best to predict, manage or avoid them.

Based on the research we do have, we often can't conclude whether a side effect could be caused by contraception or is as a result of something else, like stress or a health condition. Research into the effects of different types and amounts of progestogens and oestrogen, the interaction between them, and how they affect people differently would be so helpful. But something we talk about a lot at The Lowdown, is who would fund that research? While pharmaceutical companies have a responsibility to monitor the safety of a drug after it has been released on the market, we doubt they would investigate the non-life-threatening side effects from existing contraception, especially given the lack of investment and innovation in this space as a whole. It's also very hard to study contraception in a double-blind randomised placebo-controlled trial (a trial where neither the researchers nor the patients know whether they are getting the drug being tested or an inactive substance) because it's unethical to give participants contraception that isn't really contraception.

The Lowdown exists to fill this data gap. We gather self-reported insights on possible side effects and benefits of contraceptives to generate a better picture of how contraception can affect people in the real world. Through gathering thousands of experiences on every method and brand of contraception, we can understand which possible side effects occur most and how this varies by method and even brand. It's not a perfect science, but in the absence of more clinical research in many of these areas, it's the best we currently have, and may ever have, to help people navigate their options.

## Is it your contraception?

Two individuals can have a completely different experience with the same contraception, even if they are using the same brand. How we respond to a method likely depends on multiple factors, including age, genetics, medical background, contraceptive history and everyday lifestyle, and it's difficult to predict how someone will react.

We interact with a lot of people who ask the same very pertinent question: 'I'm feeling X – is it my contraception?' It's a good question – we all want to understand our bodies better and certainly don't want to think something we are choosing to do may unknowingly be making us feel worse. When it comes to side effects, the five areas that we get asked about the most are: mood, periods, sex drive, skin changes and weight gain. In this chapter, we dive into each of these areas to uncover what current research is out there, and what The

Lowdown's own data can tell us about how different methods are likely to impact you. Remember, not all side effects are unpleasant – some people experience improvements to their skin, lighter periods and ease of symptoms from conditions such as PMS/PMDD or PCOS, as we covered in the previous chapter.

We conducted a poll asking whether people thought their contraception side effects settled down after three months. Of the 606 responses, 73 per cent said this wasn't the case.[1] Broadly speaking, the advice is if you're still experiencing one or more of these side effects after three to six months of starting your contraception, and they're getting you down, speak to a healthcare professional about your options and whether you should switch to a different brand or method. We'll dive into exactly how you switch contraception safely later on so that you're still protected against pregnancy.

## Mood

Most of us experience changes to our mood throughout the month, and not just due to hormonal highs and lows. Work, stress, relationships and the plate-spinning of everyday life can all affect your mindset; plus, everyone's triggers are completely individual. Because of this, the impact of contraception on mood is a topic that is difficult to conduct robust, gold-standard clinical research on. Lots of the existing studies and findings are fraught with debate. At The Lowdown we've become more comfortable saying 'we don't know yet', rather than pretending we always have clear black-and-white answers to hand.

Despite many attempts to research the link between mood and contraception, the results are a mixed bag of contradictions. We know contraception can improve mood by treating conditions such as premenstrual syndrome (PMS) or premenstrual dysphoric disorder (PMDD), as well as heavy or painful periods which themselves can negatively impact mood. However, some research studies suggest that hormonal contraception can worsen mood.

A Danish study from 2016 reported that women are more likely to be started on antidepressants or diagnosed with depression for the first time if they are currently using, or have recently used, hormonal contraception.[2] While this was a huge study that looked at data from over one million women, it didn't take into account possible confounding factors (i.e. real life) and, most importantly, it did not establish that hormonal contraception *causes* depression.[3] This is the same for a study which suggested hormonal contraception may even be associated with increased risk of attempted suicide.[4]

The 2016 Danish study also suggested that progestogen-only contraceptive methods may be linked to higher rates of low mood and that non-oral forms of hormonal contraception (like the hormonal coil, patch and vaginal ring) may be linked with a higher risk of depression. Other research suggests that some particular types of progestin may be more likely to be associated with low mood, but a systematic review[5] of this stated it was limited by the risk of bias, other confounding factors and lack of a control group.[6]

Currently, there really is no clear research evidence that hormonal contraception causes depression, but we've seen from our own anecdotal data that some people do experience mood changes. At the time of writing, The Lowdown's insights on mood and contraception suggest that the hormonal coil may impact mood less than methods like the pill. Of those who reviewed the hormonal coil, 43 per cent reported no change to their mood while 31 per cent reported a negative impact on mood. This is less than the 61 per cent

## How Lowdown reviewers report that contraception affected their mood

Reviewers were asked: How do you feel this contraception has affected your moods and emotions? Reviewers could only select one option.

| | Very negatively | Somewhat negatively |
|---|---|---|
| **Combined pill** | 29% | 32% |
| **Progestogen-only pill** | 26% | 32% |
| **Hormonal coil (IUS)** | 10% | 21% |
| **Implant** | 26% | 38% |
| **Copper coil (IUD)** | 8% | 14% |
| **Injection** | 26% | 33% |
| **Patch** | 12% | 27% |
| **Vaginal ring** | 11% | 6% |

| Neutral / no change | Somewhat positively | Very positively | Don't know / can't tell |
|---|---|---|---|
| 22% | 6% | 4% | 7% |
| 25% | 7% | 3% | 7% |
| 43% | 12% | 6% | 8% |
| 23% | 4% | 1% | 8% |
| 55% | 10% | 9% | 4% |
| 27% | 3% | 4% | 7% |
| 38% | 12% | 5% | 6% |
| 72% | 11% | 0% | 0% |

Analysis of The Lowdown contraception review data July 2024. 2,466 combined pill reviews, 1,298 progestogen-only pill reviews, 767 hormonal coil (IUS) reviews, 581 implant reviews, 557 copper coil (IUD) reviews, 263 injection reviews, 97 patch reviews, 18 vaginal ring reviews.

who reported experiencing a negative impact on mood with the combined pill, and 58 per cent who reported a negative impact with the progestogen-only pill. The reason for this may be that the hormonal coil releases a lower daily dose of progestogen and acts more locally in the pelvis, compared to a method like the pill.

Not only is it hard to draw conclusions on mood from research studies, no matter how large, but there are so many different contraceptives that contain different types, doses and combinations of each hormone, including newer and older variations of them, it's hard to assess each contraceptive brand individually. Add to this that oestrogen and progestogen can interact with each other in different ways, and we have ourselves a research minefield of potential side effects. In the end, most research tends to lump all brands and types of hormonal contraceptives in the same studies, meaning it's difficult to find any specific conclusions.

While research findings vary and more studies are needed, there is some evidence to suggest that combined pills containing the newer progestogen drospirenone (pills like Yasmin, Lucette, Drovelis and Eloine) could have a more beneficial effect on mood than pills containing other progestogens.[7] Other studies suggest that using combined methods like the pill, patch or vaginal ring continuously without a break could help to reduce mood swings by avoiding the drop in hormones associated with the hormone-free break.[8] Emerging research suggests that newer pills (for example Qlaira or Zoely) containing oestrogen that is more similar to the kind naturally produced by our own bodies may also result in fewer mood side effects.[9]

What's clear is that it's important to recognise that some people will experience mood changes on hormonal contraception. If your mood isn't improving and you're concerned about your mental well-being, reach out to someone you trust or talk to your GP. You can always consider switching to something else.

**Combined pill**
Used for 3–6 months · 22 years old

★★★★★

**Yasmin pill**

This is by far the best contraceptive I've tried – before I tried Rigevidon and Gedarel 20/150, and they both gave me a very low mood almost instantly after I started taking them. Meanwhile, my mood has felt very level and similar to normal on Yasmin. My skin is pretty much the same and my periods are slightly lighter, which is a bonus. I have noticed a lower sex drive, but I am willing to take this side effect over the low mood with the other pills! This could also be due to other factors. I am glad I tried this pill and wasn't put off by the other ones I tried, as it seems to work well for me so far.

Shared on **thelowdown.com**

## Bleeding and changes to periods

From heavier and/or longer bleeding to lighter and/or more predictable (and everything in-between), there are lots of ways your bleeding pattern can be affected for better or worse with contraception. For many people, unwanted changes or problematic bleeding patterns are short lived, so it can be worth sticking to your new method for three to six months to give it a fair chance if you feel you can tolerate it.

In this section, we outline the main ways contraception can impact your periods. The most common complaint we hear about is irregular bleeding or spotting, which is more likely if you're using a progestogen-only method, but it can happen with combined contraception too. We also find that lots of people say their periods get heavier when using the copper coil, but heavy bleeding could potentially happen with any hormonal method. On the other hand, lighter bleeds are often a benefit of using combined methods or the hormonal coil. And finally, stopped periods. As hormonal contraception keeps the uterus lining thin, not having a period while on hormonal contraception is perfectly healthy and most people find this to be a positive (although for some individuals and in some cultures women may prefer to have a regular bleed). Your periods could stop while using any of the progestogen-only methods, but you can also hack it by taking your combined contraceptive back to back without a break, which is totally safe to do. Head back to pages 106–7 for a recap on what Lowdown data shows when it comes to period changes and contraception.

## Spotting on contraception

Spotting is any light bleeding (often mixed with vaginal discharge) that you may experience. Doctors may also refer to this as intermenstrual bleeding for spotting between periods if you're not using hormonal contraception, or as breakthrough bleeding if you are using combined contraception. Spotting or bleeding between periods typically occurs in the first three to six months of starting most contraceptives. It tends to settle down after a few months, but it can be a persistent pest for some.

### *What causes spotting?*

Well, the progestogen in hormonal contraception leads to changes in the lining of the uterus, making it thinner. But in turn, this can cause some bleeding, as the blood vessels in the thin uterus lining may be more fragile.

Other potential causes of spotting while on hormonal contraception include forgetting to take a pill for a day or more, or forgetting to change your ring or patch on time. Similarly, vomiting or diarrhoea can affect how well your body absorbs the pill, which can have a similar effect to when you miss a pill as you're not getting your usual dose of hormones. Smoking has also been shown to increase the likelihood of spotting or irregular bleeding.[10] Some drugs can also interfere with the effectiveness of contraceptive pills, which is why you should always check with your doctor or pharmacist before taking a new medication.

### Niddah

We do also hear from women who like having their periods at The Lowdown. This can be for a variety of reasons, but it may be interesting to know that some are deeply rooted in religious practices.

For Orthodox Jews there are religious rituals and meanings associated with a monthly period, such as the laws of niddah. Niddah (which literally translates as 'separated') is the term used to describe a woman who is having her period or has recently finished her period. Niddah includes not only the days a woman is bleeding but also a minimum of seven 'clean days' following the end of her period. During niddah, a woman is considered 'ritually impure', which means she should not participate in various activities that are considered to have religious or spiritual significance.

During niddah, a husband and wife abstain from physical intimacy. This separation usually begins when her period starts and continues until the woman has immersed in a mikveh (a ritual bath) after the clean days are completed. This marks her transition from a state of impurity to purity, allowing the resumption of marital relations.

Many Jewish women across denominations who attend the mikveh find deep spiritual or emotional enjoyment in the ritual, and the feeling of purification. For Orthodox Jewish women, the mikveh is an important religious obligation – and without niddah, there can be no need for the cleansing of the mikveh. So, contraception which stops bleeding might be seen as a loss, and the risk of irregular bleeding can disturb both sexual relations and ritual practice. This example reminds us that the impact of contraception on bleeding is not 'one size fits all'; one person's freedom might restrict someone else in ways we can't see.

*When to see your doctor about spotting*

At what stage should you consider spotting less of an annoyance and more something you should talk to a healthcare professional about? If spotting or bleeding is:

- Still occurring six months after starting a new contraceptive
- New after you've had a stable bleeding pattern for a while
- Occurring regularly after sex
- Combined with discharge, especially if there's an unpleasant smell
- Occurring after a change in sexual partner

- Heavy (soaking a pad or tampon hourly for more than two hours)
- Generally concerning you or if you have any other symptoms you're worried about.

In some cases, spotting or bleeding while on hormonal contraception can suggest signs of an underlying health condition, sexually transmitted infection (STI), pregnancy, or it may even be the result of things like vaginal dryness.

The first two things you especially need to check for if you have new bleeding or a change in bleeding pattern are sexually transmitted infections and pregnancy. If you have an STI, this can lead to irritation and inflammation of the uterus or cervix, which can cause bleeding. Sometimes light bleeding or spotting can occur when a fertilised egg implants into the lining of the uterus as a pregnancy starts. It can also occur in early pregnancy and be a sign of early pregnancy complications and pregnancy loss. If you've been using your contraception correctly the chance of this is small but a pregnancy test is usually advised, especially if your bleeding is new or the pattern has changed.

If you notice any unusual symptoms alongside spotting, like pain or itching, speak to your GP. They will ensure you're tested for STIs and pregnancy, check your cervical screening is up to date and examine you to confirm there are no changes to the cervix, vagina or pelvic anatomy that may be causing bleeding.

### *Which types of contraception are most likely to cause spotting?*

Overall, combined hormonal contraception (the combined pill, patch or vaginal ring) is often very good at controlling bleeding. Most users of combined contraception will only experience bleeding if they choose to have the four to seven day pill-free break in which they will likely experience a light, predictable withdrawal bleed. However, you also have the freedom to choose to have fewer bleeds, or none at all, by using combined methods without a break. These methods can cause spotting for some people, especially in the first month and up to three months for around 20 per cent of people who use them.[11] Of course, everyone is different, and it's not all down to hormones. For instance, our data shows that 21 per cent of people using the copper coil (IUD) also experienced spotting or irregular bleeding.[12]

Spotting or irregular bleeding on combined contraception, also known as breakthrough bleeding, can be annoying and unpredictable. Changing to a different combined pill with a higher oestrogen dose,[13] or switching to the vaginal ring, which has been shown to be associated with less unscheduled bleeding,[14] may help to make breakthrough bleeding more manageable.

Conversely, progestogen-only methods can all have a variable effect on your cycle, making you much less in control of when and how much you bleed. Although some people find that they don't bleed at all, studies show that progestogen-only contraceptives (the progestogen-only pill, implant, injection and hormonal coil) are the most likely to cause spotting. Research evidence suggests the implant is most likely to cause no periods or infrequent bleeds, however around 20 per cent of people using the implant experience prolonged episodes of bleeding of fourteen days or longer, and less than 10 per cent will experience frequent spotting.[15] We compared this to The Lowdown review data, which shows 65 per cent of users of the implant reported irregular bleeding or spotting.[16] The bleeding pattern you have in the first three months of using the implant is generally a good predictor of what your bleeds will be like for the time you use it, which can be for up to three years. If you have prolonged or frequent bleeding, there is still a 50 per cent chance that this pattern will improve, but it may take until the second year of use.[17]

Desogestrel and drospirenone-based progestogen-only pills have similar spotting rates to the implant and stop periods altogether in up to 30 per cent of users. If you use an older type of progestogen-only pill (Noriday or Norgeston), spotting is more likely than with new pills.[18]

On the injection, bleeding issues including spotting, bleeding for over fourteen days or heavy bleeding are common initially, but after twelve months of use 50 per cent of users won't have any bleeding at all.[19] Our data suggests that for well over half of our users, the injection stopped their periods (70 per cent). Comparatively, only 13 per cent reported irregular periods, and 13 per cent said they had spotting or breakthrough bleeding.[20]

**Injection**
Used for 5–8 years 25 years old

★★★★☆

**Depo-Provera injection**

Was on Depo aged sixteen to twenty-two and I only came off it after concerns about long-term effects (i.e. osteoporosis). At first, I had about three to six months of daily spotting, which stopped after a nurse practitioner suggested I take my depo on week 11 instead of week 12. It's great because it doesn't interfere with daily life, and the only major con after the breakthrough bleeding was dryness and spotting after sex. Had some pain for a day after on the injection site and leg occasionally but nothing too painful.

Shared on **thelowdown.com**

*How to manage spotting*

Our top tips to minimise spotting or irregular bleeding in the first few months include taking your pill at a similar time each day. If you're taking any new medications, and if you experience vomiting or diarrhoea that you think might be affecting your ability to absorb the pill, talk to your doctor or pharmacist. If you use the implant, injection or hormonal coil, your GP may suggest taking the combined (if you're eligible) or desogestrel-based pill alongside for three months to see if this helps.

While there's currently no evidence to suggest that taking two desogestrel progestogen-only pills a day will help control bleeding, in reality some practitioners do suggest trying a double dose.[21] This is called prescribing something 'off licence', because while it can have a desired effect, it's not part of a medication's intended use for which it was originally licensed, and often there is no specific related research. Anecdotally it can work for some people, and it can be worth a try, but the downside is that it may increase side effects like acne, bloating and mood changes, so it's not always an ideal tactic if you're sensitive to progestogen. Like continuous pill taking, this is another example of 'off-licence' use which is totally safe to do.

**Muslim prayer and bleeding side effects**

The following explanation is thanks to our fabulous Lowdown clinical lead Dr Zaakira Mahomed.

'The menstrual period in Islam is called Haydh. This is defined as any regular bleed that lasts between three and ten days. In this time a woman is unable to pray the obligatory five daily prayers, fast or read the Quran. However, she is encouraged to engage in other forms of worship. Any bleeding outside of Haydh if it is within fifteen days is known as Istihaadha and has its own set of rules. Spotting or bleeding due to contraception will fall under this category. During the Haydh period, a woman should abstain from sexual intercourse with her husband but other forms of intimacy and closeness are still acceptable. When the period of Haydh is finished a woman must take a Ghusl (ritual bath) to cleanse herself. Thereafter, praying, fasting and intercourse may resume. Any missed fasts will need to be made up at a later date but prayers do not need to be compensated for. In some cultures, periods can be seen as unclean but in Islam, periods are seen as a natural process. Women who are on their periods are encouraged to rest and religious obligations are relaxed so they do not become a source of undue hardship. It allows Muslim women to honour their faith while respecting their physical and emotional well-being, but may mean irregular or unpredictable bleeds are troublesome for some Muslim women.'

## Heavier periods

The non-hormonal copper coil (IUD) can be associated with longer, heavier and more painful periods, so it's often best to avoid this method if you already have these symptoms. We're not sure why this happens, but it's thought to be down to prostaglandin release and mild inflammation caused by copper released into the uterus – which is essential to immobilise any sneaky sperm. Thankfully, these changes can improve after six to twelve months,[22] but anecdotally we do hear from some people who find these side effects last until they have the copper coil removed.

**Copper coil (IUD)**
Used for 18 months to 3 years 39 years old

★★★☆☆

**Copper coil (IUD)**
Pros – non hormonal, the placement doesn't cause me discomfort, I can forget about it and for three years it hasn't caused me any concern on unwanted pregnancies. Cons – the doctor I had to insert the coil was amazing, and it was no more discomfort than a smear, however the two to three days following I was in a lot of pain. It did settle. I suffered with BV [bacterial vaginosis] two/three times while my body became used to the coil in my body. Vaginal dryness is the biggest thing for me, which I've never experienced before and, lastly, longer heavier periods. The heavy side has taken two years to settle down, the random cramps and spotting has settled and is less frequent and my period lasts longer. Not completely ideal for me but currently, with the pros of protection and being non hormonal, it's the best option for me.

Shared on **thelowdown.com**

## Lighter and stopped periods

When it comes to contraception that causes lighter periods, the clear frontrunner from The Lowdown's review data is the combined pill. We've outlined how progestogen thins the uterus lining to prevent pregnancy, which impacts bleeding in different ways. Often, it results in lighter withdrawal bleeds on the hormone-free break, compared to the bleeding you'd likely experience during a 'normal' period. Eventually for some people, the uterus lining becomes so thin that bleeding stops completely. So if you use the combined pill, patch or ring and take your hormone-free break, it's normal to bleed lightly during this time, or not bleed at all. As we've previously mentioned, you can also skip your bleed completely by using it continuously without any scheduled breaks for as many months as you want.

Progestogen-only contraception methods (progestogen-only pill, injection, implant and hormonal coil) can all have a variable effect on your cycle. With all of these options there is no hormone-free break (apart from the drospirenone-containing pill Slynd) to decide whether you have a bleed or not and unscheduled bleeding is a common side effect, meaning you're not in control of when and how much you bleed. However, it's common that lots of people using these methods have no bleeding at all (what doctors call 'amenorrhoea'), but this varies between each method. Research evidence suggests that generally after twelve months, 20–30 per cent of people using the desogestrel-based progestogen-only pill,[23] 50 per cent using the contraceptive injection and 20 per cent of people using the implant will not bleed at all.[24]

When it comes to stopping periods altogether, Lowdown users report that the injection is the best contraceptive for this, with 70 per cent of people reporting this as the main side effect. In comparison, 45 per cent of Lowdown users say that their periods stopped altogether when using the progestogen-only pill.[25]

With all types of hormonal coil, spotting is common in the first three to six months of having it fitted. But once you get past this, research has shown that for the Mirena, Levosert or Benilexa brands of hormonal coil, around 40 per cent of users will have no periods in the long run.[26] In comparison, lower dose hormonal coils, like the Jaydess, may not control bleeding or spotting as successfully, but around one in eight Jaydess users and one in four Kyleena users still find they have no periods at all.[27] At The Lowdown, we found that 48 per cent of people said that the hormonal coil stopped their periods, and 25 per cent said they became lighter.[28] When we break this down by each brand, 53 per cent reported that the Mirena coil stopped their periods and 57 per cent of Levosert users said their periods got lighter. Comparatively, only 36 per cent of Jaydess and 36 per cent of Kyleena users said their periods stopped completely.[29]

## Sex drive

Having a high or low sex drive is used to describe interest in sex or sexual activity. It's completely normal for your sex drive, also referred to as libido, to fluctuate throughout life – no one can be horny all the time. There are tons of things that can impact your sex drive for days, weeks or months at a time. From daily life stresses to big life changes: think moving house, changing job, having kids, changes to your mental and physical health, medications you use, menopause, and so on. There is no concrete evidence that hormonal contraception affects sex drive; however, other side effects of hormonal contraception, such as vaginal dryness, may indirectly affect libido. And the irony isn't lost on us that lots of us use hormonal contraception to prevent pregnancy only then to not feel like having sex. Make it make sense, please.

From what little research there is into sex drive, there has been mixed results about whether contraception can directly affect libido. However, it is a frequently reported side effect at The Lowdown. A review looking at all of the evidence surrounding combined contraception and libido up to 2012 found that a small number of women experienced an increase or decrease in libido, while the majority of participants across studies experienced no changes to their sexual desire at all.[30] Another review found no consistent pattern between having a higher or lower sex drive either – in fact, most experienced no change whatsoever.[31] The researchers here suggest that any changes might be due to a complex interaction of psychological, social and biological effects, which are really difficult to tease apart.

Research on combined hormonal contraception suggests that taking it continuously without a break may actually be better for sex drive than having regular breaks.[32] However, other research has suggested that a continuous contraception regimen could worsen the quality of a woman's sexual life before causing an improvement.[33] See what we mean about a mixed bag? Specifically looking at the role of oestrogen and sex drive changes, it's interesting to see some research has found that combined hormonal contraceptives containing lower levels of oestrogen might have a better effect on sex drive than ones containing higher doses.[34] Plus, participants who used a newer, low-dose combined pill with a shorter pill-free break also generally saw improved sex drive over time. Again, though, this appears to affect only a small number of users.

Combined hormonal contraception has also been found to lower the levels of testosterone in the body, and there is some evidence to suggest that testosterone can influence libido in women and people assigned female at birth.[35] One study, looking at women aged eighteen to thirty-five, found that testosterone decreased while using combined hormonal contraception but it had no significant impact on sex drive.[36] It's thought that the effect of testosterone on libido could be affected by the sensitivity of an individual's androgen receptors (the receptors in the brain that bind testosterone).

## How Lowdown reviewers reported contraception changed their sex drive

Reviewers were asked: Have you noticed any changes to your sex drive while using this contraception? Reviewers could select one option.

| | Decreased sex drive |
|---|---|
| **Combined pill** | 47% |
| **Progestogen-only pill** | 51% |
| **Hormonal coil (IUS)** | 28% |
| **Implant** | 50% |
| **Copper coil (IUD)** | 12% |
| **Injection** | 58% |
| **Fertility awareness methods** | 0% |
| **Patch** | 19% |
| **Male condom** | 9% |
| **Vaginal ring** | 28% |

| **Increased sex drive** | **No change** | **Don't know** |
|---|---|---|
| 7% | 31% | 15% |
| 8% | 31% | 10% |
| 10% | 47% | 15% |
| 6% | 29% | 15% |
| 16% | 63% | 9% |
| 5% | 27% | 10% |
| 47% | 45% | 8% |
| 13% | 52% | 16% |
| 9% | 73% | 9% |
| 6% | 44% | 22% |

Analysis of The Lowdown contraception review data July 2024. 2,466 combined pill reviews, 1,298 progestogen-only pill reviews, 767 hormonal coil (IUS) reviews, 581 implant reviews, 557 copper coil (IUD) reviews, 263 injection reviews, 115 fertility awareness methods reviews, 97 patch reviews, 23 male condom reviews, 18 vaginal ring reviews.

Essentially, whether or not your libido is affected by changing levels of testosterone could just be down to your unique biology.

At the time of writing, The Lowdown's data shows that 47 per cent of combined pill users found that their sex drive decreased (we only have a small number of reviews for the ring and the patch which are less widely used).[37] It's important to note that we have a lot more reviews for the combined pill than the ring and the patch, as it's more widely used.

The effects of progestogen-only contraception on libido aren't well studied, but the current evidence suggests that it doesn't have a negative impact on sex drive overall, and there's no significant link.[38] However, 58 per cent of injection users, 51 per cent of progestogen-only pill users, 50 per cent of implant users and 28 per cent of hormonal coil users reported decreased sex drive on The Lowdown. Nearly half (47 per cent) of the people who reviewed the hormonal coil reported no changes.[39] But why are so many people who come to The Lowdown reporting these changes in sex drive, if all the evidence points to no significant links?

Well, when it comes to *indirectly* affecting sex drive there's a possibility that other side effects of contraception could have a knock-on effect. For instance, we know that users of the progestogen-only pill have higher rates of symptoms such as vaginal dryness, low mood or irregular bleeding, which could all have an impact. Similarly, the non-hormonal copper coil can cause increased or prolonged bleeding and painful cramps, which aren't usually known for their sex appeal. On the flip side of this, your hormonal contraceptive might have reduced your bleeding, cleared up your skin or helped you manage mood swings, which could all indirectly boost your sex drive too.

**Hormonal coil (IUS)**
Used for 5–8 years    41years old

★★★★☆

**Mirena coil**

Much lighter periods. Had some emotional times and very low sex drive but unsure if that was the IUD or post-pregnancy life.

Shared on **thelowdown.com**

As sex drive is influenced by many different factors, switching contraception is only one part of addressing an issue with this. For instance, if you're experiencing vaginal dryness and it's putting a downer on your sex drive, you could try using lubricant during sex, vaginal moisturisers or you could be prescribed vaginal oestrogen cream. If you're looking for more support around problems with sex itself, a pelvic health physiotherapist can help with gynaecological conditions that cause pain during sex, or seeing a sex therapist to work through your emotional or mental struggles with sex drive could help. Reaching out to your GP if you're constantly feeling low is also a good idea. If after three to six months of using a contraceptive, your sex drive still doesn't return to what was normal for you before you started, then speak to your healthcare professional about options and whether to consider switching your method.

**Q:** I've lost my sex drive and don't want to change my contraception, what can I do to increase it?

We asked The Lowdown's resident Sex and Relationships coach, Lucy Rowett, to answer this one:

**A:** 'Your libido will always wax and wane throughout your life and you should expect it. Lots of people don't know that your libido and desire are not the same thing. While libido is a physical or emotional urge, desire encompasses thoughts, emotions and overall well-being.

'To nurture desire, consider life stressors and self-care: ensure proper nutrition, hydration, sunlight, movement, sleep and relaxation. These basics, when neglected, can stress the body and diminish libido. Identify what specifically turns you on and off, and take practical steps to enhance your sexual environment and mood.

'Proactively create conditions for desire. Explore erotica, including ethical and feminist porn, and engage in self-pleasuring. Regular masturbation can increase sexual desire by rewiring neural pathways. Sensual movement or dancing can boost body confidence, blood flow to the pelvis and overall mood, making you feel sexy for yourself.

'Evaluate if you genuinely enjoy the sex you're having. If not, identify and communicate your needs, ensuring your sexual experiences are fulfilling. Use lube if experiencing vaginal dryness. Ultimately, reclaiming libido involves finding pleasure, rediscovering your sexy self and feeling good in your body.'

## Skin changes

Acne is a really common skin condition. Ninety-five per cent of people between the ages of eleven and thirty will have it at some point,[40] but it can affect anyone well into adulthood. While there's plenty of advice and research out there on how to manage acne through medications, dermatological treatments and sometimes diet and lifestyle changes, we love to talk about our area of expertise: hormonal changes. In general, combined methods tend to improve acne over time, while

**Progestogen only/mini pill**
Used for 8+ years 27 years old

★★★★☆

**Desogestrel pill**

This is an easy and quick contraception method which I have found really beneficial to me personally. My periods have now essentially stopped, with very irregular periods now being the norm with my last period being over a year ago. Because of that, when I get a period it is only a few days at a time, whereas before they would sometimes last over two weeks. Menstrual pain such as cramps, lower back pain etc. are also a lot more controlled. I still get these every month or two but they don't last for long and the pain has decreased massively, although I do get breast tenderness more than I used to pre-pill. The downsides, though, do include acne, which has had periods of improving/getting worse, and weight gain. Overall, though, I like the ease of this (mine is the 12-hour mini pill) compared to other options out there.

Shared on **thelowdown.com**

progestogen-only contraception might lead to spots or worsen acne in some people. The Lowdown's insights at the time of writing show that 45 per cent of combined pill users reported improved skin, whereas 47 per cent of progestogen-only pill reviewers reported no change to their skin and 28 per cent reported that they felt it made their skin worse.[41]

Despite some evidence to suggest that certain progestogens in combined pills can improve acne, the very limited research we have means an association between the progestogen-only pill and acne can't be confirmed, but we do know that some people find taking the progestogen-only pill makes their skin worse or triggers acne.[42] This could be because the synthetic progestogen in the progestogen-only pill may bind to androgen receptors in the body causing your skin to produce more of that pore-clogging sebum. The same applies for the contraceptive injection or implant. However, on The Lowdown only 18 per cent of implant users and 22 per cent of injection users reported worse skin.[43]

Overall, research is too limited to establish if the hormonal coil causes acne. The amount of progestogen in the coil is much lower than that found in other progestogen-only contraceptives, so theoretically there may be less of a noticeable impact on the skin. Although this hasn't been proven in research, and our own data suggests that it is similar to other progestogen-only methods, as 23 per cent of Lowdown users said their skin got worse when using the hormonal coil.[44]

If you're struggling with acne and decide to use isotretinoin therapy as treatment (this can come under different brand names, like Roaccutane), there's a small risk that your contraceptive pill could be less effective.[45] Your healthcare professional should talk you through your contraceptive options while using this kind of acne treatment; it's very important to avoid pregnancy given that isotretinoin is dangerous for growing foetuses. They might suggest using a LARC method, like the injection or implant, because of its high effectiveness.

## Weight gain

We all naturally gain weight with age and many lifestyle factors can influence weight fluctuation. This can be due to things like diet, movement levels, sleep quality, and even how much stress we're under. Just like mood and sex drive, this can make it difficult for research to gain an accurate measure of how much contraception impacts weight.

If you have a bigger body, it can feel like all you hear when deciding on a contraceptive is the methods that you can't use, because of the associated health risks of using combined hormonal contraception when you have a higher BMI (see Chapter 6 on health risks). We know that BMI is a rubbish assessment of individual wellness or health. It was originally developed to look at population not individual health, is based on data from white males (common theme here), doesn't take into account how much fat or muscle you have or how this is distributed, and doesn't account for variations in our bone density and bodily structure. It's frustratingly flawed, but nevertheless all health guidelines currently use it.

We've heard of women dreading going to their contraception review appointments because they really don't want to be weighed, adding a layer of upset to what's already a highly personal experience for some. We'll look more closely at the associated risks in the next chapter, but going into your appointment with prior knowledge of what methods are better suited to you if you have a higher BMI, i.e. most of the progestogen-only methods or non-hormonal methods, will help you go into your consultation more empowered to make your own choice.

For most methods of hormonal contraception, research has not identified a formal link to weight gain, that is except for the injection. Experiencing weight gain may be more likely if you start to use the injection under the age of eighteen and your BMI is over 30, which sounds alarming, but in reality, most people don't gain weight while using the injection.[46] We also know that if you gain more than 5 per cent of your body weight within six months of starting the injection, you may be more likely to continue gaining weight.[47] At the time of writing, 49 per cent of people using the injection told The Lowdown that they had gained weight; the highest percentage

**Injection**
Used for 18 months to 3 years 19 years old

★★★★☆

**Depo-Provera injection**

Overall one of the best contraceptives I've tried and I've tried some form of each. Started using to help with endo-associated pain and heavy periods. It completely stopped my periods, other than the occasional spotting towards the end of the twelve weeks after injection. I found it had no long term impact on my moods and very few side effects in general and improved my skin. Really handy only having to get it every twelve weeks rather than take a pill every day. Only downfalls are for about a week after the first two injections I was very teary and hungry all the time, but this stopped once I got used to it. It also had an impact on sex drive and caused weight gain during the whole time I was on it.

Shared on **thelowdown.com**

of all the contraceptive users. Thirty-five per cent reported no change in weight, and 4 per cent reported weight loss.[48] One reason for perceived weight gain while using combined contraception might be water retention. Oestrogen and progesterone affect the way our kidneys produce certain proteins, which can impact how the body regulates water and cause an increase in the fluid within the body's tissues. This kind of water retention can also happen naturally just before your period, causing that ever-so-familiar puffy 'bleurgh' feeling. Combined pills which contain newer progestins such as drospirenone have properties which mean they are less likely to cause water retention than others.[49]

Research has (again) found limited evidence of changes in weight while using other progestogen-only contraceptives, and water retention is less likely to happen with newer progestogens in certain pill brands.[50] Lowdown users were pretty evenly split on this one: at the time of writing 44 per cent of those using the progestogen-only pill reported no change in their weight, with 36 per cent saying they'd gained weight and 5 per cent saying they'd seen a decrease in weight. With the hormonal coil, 59 per cent reported no change in their weight, 18 per cent experienced weight gain and 5 per cent said they had weight loss. Implant users reported a similar experience to those on the progestogen-only pill, with 38 per cent reporting no change in their weight, 41 per cent reporting an increase and 3 per cent noticing weight loss.[51]

But what about combined methods? One study has hypothesised that oestrogen may promote fat storage.[52] However, after much debate, there is no proof that combined hormonal contraception causes weight gain. In fact, a review of available research in 2014 found no causal link between combined hormonal contraception and weight gain.[53] Despite what the research says, we know that anecdotally

**Patch**
Used for 6–12 months 26 years old

★★★☆☆

**Evra patch**

The patch was OK. I definitely preferred it to taking a pill every day but still had the issue of remembering when I had to put the new one on. My biggest issue with it was that as it's sticky, it would get very dirty, very quickly either from sweat, clothes lint or general dirt and would start to lose its stickiness and did fall off a couple of times. I noticed quite a bit of weight gain as well as very enlarged breasts and there was an obvious loss of sex drive. I'm unsure I would use it again.

Shared on **thelowdown.com**

weight comes up in our reported side effects time and again. Of those who reviewed the combined pill at The Lowdown 48 per cent reported no change in weight, while 30 per cent said they had gained weight and 4 per cent said that they had lost weight. For the patch, 48 per cent of users reported no change, 26 per cent reported weight gain and 4 per cent said that they had lost weight. The vaginal ring seems to have the highest percentage of users reporting more stability in their weight, with 72 per cent of users reporting no change, 11 per cent reporting weight gain and 6 per cent reporting weight loss.[54]

Women of reproductive age tend to gain weight over time, whether they're using contraception or not.[55] However, if weight gain is something you struggle with or are worried about, particularly if you have PCOS, talk your options through with your healthcare professional before switching. Before writing off your contraception completely, it's also worth thinking about any recent changes you might have had to your lifestyle: whether your diet has changed, your alcohol intake has increased, you're not as active as you used to be, or if you're taking any other medications that have weight gain as a possible side effect. If you haven't noticed any changes to your routine, or you just aren't sure, your GP is there to help.

## Other common side effects

Of course, there are other side effects that pop up quite a lot in our research. We couldn't list them all in this chapter, but there are four more that definitely deserve a shout out.

- **Bigger boobs and painful boobs** There are thousands of contraception experiences on The Lowdown and around half of them are for a type of pill. Staggeringly, at the time of writing over 50 per cent of users of both types of pill reported tender breasts, and 41–47 per cent said that their boobs got bigger on the pill.[56] The hormones in contraception can cause water retention and changes to breast tissue. Breast tenderness usually improves within a few months of starting to take the pill. If your breasts are larger because you're experiencing water retention, you might notice that they return to normal during your pill-free break (if you have one). Keeping a diary for a couple of months may help with this. If you carry on taking the pill, or stop taking it altogether, your boobs should go back to their normal size.
- **Headaches and migraines** Did you know that from puberty onwards, women are prone to more migraines than men? This might provide a clue to the link between migraines

**Implant**
Used for 6–12 months 26 years old

★★☆☆☆

**Nexplanon implant**

My experience with the implant started off really well, my period disappeared! But then it came back with a vengeance alongside headaches, period cramps and loss of sex drive. I started feeling like myself when I came off it.

Shared on **thelowdown.com**

and hormones, although clinical evidence is too limited to demonstrate that hormonal contraception actually causes headaches or migraines.[57] If you've ever read the back of the pill packet, headaches are listed as a side effect, although in many cases they tend to lessen over time and the majority of people who share their experience on The Lowdown report that they don't get headaches with their contraception. If you experience headaches associated with your period or in the days just before, this may be due to the drop in oestrogen and the release of prostaglandins (that cause cramping). Hormonal contraception that stops you ovulating or stops your periods may improve this. For those taking combined contraception the pill-free break can replicate this drop in oestrogen, so headaches may be worse. Taking combined contraception continuously can help avoid these headaches. The difference between a headache and a migraine can be very subtle, and it's important to speak to a healthcare professional to get the right diagnosis. There are small increased risks associated with combined contraception for migraine sufferers, especially those who experience what's known as an aura with their migraines. We take a look at this in the next chapter.

• **Digestive issues** Oestrogen can cause nausea, or make it worse if you already experience it. This is especially true when you first start taking the pill, and for some people the nausea can pass after a few months of taking the pill – or be minimised by taking it at night or with food. These issues are somewhat reflected in our own data, as 30 per cent of combined pill reviewers and 24 per cent of progestogen-only pill reviewers reported nausea or vomiting.[58] However, remember a common cause of nausea is pregnancy, so if this is a new symptom consider doing a pregnancy test. If you want to keep taking a pill, you may want to opt for a brand with a lower dose of oestrogen or try a progestogen-only or non-hormonal contraceptive option.

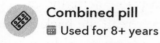

**Combined pill**
Used for 8+ years 27 years old

★★★★★

**Lizinna pill**

Very few side effects other than a bit of breast tenderness and nausea in the first couple of months. Since then I've had much lighter periods and it helped with breakouts.

Shared on **thelowdown.com**

Oestrogen and progestogen can also slow down the movement of your gut; this could mean bloating, constipation and discomfort may be more likely. There is also a relationship between the oestrogen we produce and the good bacteria that live in our gut (microbiome), so it's plausible that this could also be affected by oestrogen in the pill, but we have no research evidence for this yet.

If you often experience digestive issues due to inflammatory bowel disease, irritable bowel syndrome or anything else – opting for a method of contraception that doesn't go through your digestive system can reduce any impact the hormones may have on your digestion, and it can be comforting to know the effectiveness of the contraception won't be affected by vomiting or diarrhoea.

- **Vaginal dryness** About 20 per cent of pre-menopausal women in the UK suffer from vaginal dryness,[59] and this increases during perimenopause (the time leading up to your periods stopping completely) when your natural oestrogen levels start to decline. Oestrogen is the hormone responsible for keeping your vagina and vulva well lubed, FYI.

**Vaginal ring**
Used for 18 months to 3 years · 29 years old

★★★★☆

**NuvaRing**

I really loved using the ring, compared to the pill the side effects were minimal and absolutely no bother in remembering it. Unfortunately, my doctor just made me come off it as my blood pressure has steadily gone up over three years of using it. I did experience loss of sex drive, and vaginal dryness which led to thrush infections. But no changes in mood or skin!

Shared on **thelowdown.com**

We know that hormonal contraceptive methods have been linked to increased vaginal dryness.[60] As it stands 38–39 per cent of Lowdown users said they experienced vaginal dryness while using the combined pill, progestogen-only pill or implant, while 42 per cent said they experienced vaginal dryness whilst using the injection.[61] Off licence, some healthcare professionals may prescribe vaginal oestrogens, which can be excellent at improving lubrication.

No one should have to put up with feeling rubbish as a result of contraception, so if you're not getting along with yours, doing your research before speaking to your doctor, nurse or pharmacist about other options will really help you make the most of a short appointment time.

# 6

# Health risks (but don't panic!)

We're swamped with news stories about ways to live longer, healthier lives: gut-happy diets to follow, exercise plans to incorporate and the perfect amount of deep sleep to help us live to 100. On the other side of the coin, column inches are filled with stories about risks to our well-being, from exposure to toxins and lifestyle choices, through to our genetics. Sometimes the research quoted is difficult to understand or contradicts medical advice that has come before. Other times elements of the research are misquoted or relayed out of context for extra clicks. Statements around our increased risk of developing certain illnesses can sound really scary and it's easy to become consumed in hypothetical risk statistics without understanding what it actually means for us.

Like every medication, contraception carries benefits and risks. We're all comfortable with different levels of risk in our everyday life and there is no one 'right' way when it comes to balancing risk versus reward. So, in this chapter, we're going to look at the main risks associated with taking contraception – understanding these will help you make an informed decision about the contraception you choose (or choose not) to use.

In order to make sense of the complex subject of risk,

we'll first take a look at how doctors explain it and how we interpret it. Then let's figure out how the data applies to us as individuals, and whether we need to worry about it. When we hear scaremongering concerning hormonal contraception, it's often around the risks people (rightly or often wrongly) associate with it. We aim to tackle these misconceptions head-on and look at what the evidence says and how contraception can also protect against certain cancers and conditions. In fact, for most people, the advantages of hormonal contraception far outweigh the risks.

## Understanding risk

From over-the-counter treatments like paracetamol or herbal remedies to vaccines and other life-saving medicines, there are potential risks from all medications. When you are prescribed hormonal contraception, your GP, nurse or pharmacist should discuss the risks with you. It can be challenging to explain medical risk to patients because human nature struggles to comprehend risk as a concept. We humans don't do well with uncertainty either, so it's no wonder we find risk tricky.

Understanding your personal risk when taking contraception is important. You can then weigh the risks against the benefits contraception offers to see if it's worth it for you. Here are some things to keep in mind to help you think about risk.

- **'Absolute' and 'relative' risk** Absolute risk is the term used to describe the chance of developing a condition. It is often spoken about in different ways, such as, 'You have a 1 in 10 risk of developing . . .' or, 'You have a 10 per cent risk of developing . . .' both of which mean the same thing. If you're told you have a 10 per cent chance of developing an illness, that can feel quite abstract.

Absolute risk can be used to show the chance of developing a condition in different groups. For example, 'There is a 1 in 10 risk of developing a condition in non smokers and a 3 in 10 risk of developing the same condition in smokers.' Relative risk, on the other hand, *compares* the risk between two different groups. For example, 'Your risk of developing breast cancer increases if you regularly drink alcohol.' This statement explains how one group of people (those who regularly drink alcohol) are more likely to develop breast cancer than another group (those who don't drink alcohol).

Using relative risk can make the numbers look pretty shocking. For example, if you have a baseline 1 in 100,000 risk of developing an illness, but a study shows those who exercise less have a 2 in 100,000 risk of developing the same illness, the relative increase in risk here is 100 per cent, or we could say the risk doubles for those who exercise less, but the absolute increase in risk of 1 more person in 100,000 developing the illness is actually a very small number. Relative risk is often misquoted from studies as it makes clickbait headlines, but without the absolute risk numbers it tells us nothing of the actual likelihood of something happening. Throughout this chapter we'll refer back to absolute and relative risk.

A favourite analogy on relative risk that we use is that it's like saying you finished third in your age group in a sporting event, without telling people that there were only three people in that sporting event in your age group. Without that context, it's not clear that you finished last in the race!

- **Keeping perspective** It can sound alarming to hear that your risk of developing certain conditions or side effects can increase when you use particular contraceptives. The reality is that sometimes the numbers behind these stats are still very low. It's important to keep in mind how common a condition is in the first place as while the risk may have gone up slightly, it's still statistically unlikely you will develop the illness in question.

• **Language** The language used to describe risk can affect how we perceive it. How we, as individuals, interpret risk varies too – two people might emerge from a medical appointment with a different interpretation of what the doctor has told them. Some healthcare professionals are naturally better than others at explaining medical information and risks to their patients. There has been some focus in recent years on doctors using clear, simple language to help patients process what they're saying (which is especially important if you've been given overwhelming news).

If you're not a numbers person, interpreting data that uses percentages, decimals and fractions can be even tougher. Ask your doctor if they can explain the risks in another way, such as signposting you to some graphs or charts (visual people often do better with these).

Some other things to bear in mind when you are making a decision regarding the risks around your contraceptive method include . . .

• **Weighing up risk versus benefit** When assessing the risk of hormonal contraception, it's important to balance it against the potential benefits and risk of pregnancy; this is a key concept so read carefully. Spoiler alert – pregnancy is a risky business, probably one of the riskiest things a woman can do in her lifetime. Pregnancy causes significant changes in the body which lead to an increased risk of developing blood clots, high blood pressure and conditions like pre-eclampsia and gestational diabetes. Potential complications during delivery, such as excessive bleeding or the need for emergency surgery, also contribute to the risk. Additionally, pregnancy can impact mental health, leading to issues like postpartum depression. For most people, pregnancy risks far outweigh the risks associated with contraception. Your healthcare professional is always balancing the impact of a contraceptive method against the inherent risks of an unintended pregnancy.

Your personal circumstances matter too; for example, what are the alternatives? If using a contraceptive isn't all that essential to your day-to-day, you may be more willing to explore alternatives that you only use when you have sex, like condoms. Contraceptives also have medical benefits that should be taken into account. From everyday positives like helping with symptoms of PMS, painful and/or heavy periods and acne, to managing conditions like PCOS and endometriosis, and to having a protective effect against certain cancers, many feel the rewards, on balance, are worth the small risks.

- **Subjectivity** There's an element of subjectivity around risk which may also change with your circumstances and throughout your life. When it comes to choosing one type of contraception over another, for one person, for example, the 'risk' of unplanned pregnancy may not be too big a deal, while for another, the consequences will be devastating.
- **Personal preferences** We all hold values, and different things are important to different people. This means our approach to weighing up risk versus benefit may well differ from our partner, friend or family member. Assessing risk is something we instinctively do every day, much of it subconsciously, like crossing a road. Human nature varies in our comfort level with risk, so only you can make a decision about what you're OK with.

## Typical risk assessments your doctor or healthcare professional will make before prescribing hormonal contraception

Your healthcare professional will assess your risk factors before prescribing contraception (or any other medication). They'll take into account your personal medical history, including any other medication you're taking or relevant lifestyle factors, and they'll also ask about your family medical history. If you are prescribed combined contraception, you will have an annual review, which includes a blood pressure check, as well as reassessing your risk and checking for any new medical conditions.

• **Assessing risk** Healthcare professionals in the UK use a huge document of guidelines from the FSRH that's nearly 200 pages long to help assess risk. This is called the UK Medical Eligibility Criteria, UKMEC for short.[1] In this document, the risk of using contraceptive methods is broken down into four levels which are applied to a whole range of medical conditions or lifestyle factors. To simplify things, we have summarised those levels as follows:

- Level 1 means crack on, the contraceptive method is considered safe to use.
- Level 2 means the advantages of using the contraceptive method outweigh any associated risks.
- Level 3 means that the risks associated with the contraceptive now generally outweigh the benefits, so in these scenarios the contraceptive can only be used with specialist input.
- Level 4 means absolutely no way; it's far too risky for you to take this method of contraception.

So now let's look at why these potential risks are at the forefront of a healthcare professional's mind when prescribing hormonal contraception.

## How can contraception affect my health?

### Cancer

Cancer is a subject no one wants to linger over, though it is one people (rightly) want to know more about when they are weighing up their contraceptive options, and it's important we're clued up about our individual risk.

There are so many factors that can increase the risk of getting cancer, such as genetics and lifestyle. While we can't do anything about the genes we've inherited, we can focus on lifestyle practices that put us in everyday good health and may help protect against cancer. The top-line tips are fairly common sense: maintain a healthy weight, keep fit, enjoy a varied and balanced diet, don't smoke and limit alcohol. Think of these five recommendations as being on the 'greatest hits' album of lifestyle choices to improve your health by doctors everywhere: they pop up a lot.

Now for the lowdown on what we know about different types of cancers and how they're impacted by both combined and progestogen-only contraception. We'll look at how contraception can slightly increase and slightly decrease our risk of getting certain types of cancer. It's worth noting, too, that 'cancer' is a catch-all term to describe really varied diseases and outcomes. The good news is that medical advancements are making diagnosis, treatment and outcomes more and more effective than in previous generations.

*Breast cancer*

We've known for some time that combined methods (those that contain both oestrogen and progestogen) slightly increase the risk of breast cancer. A study[2] has found that the amounts and types of oestrogen and progestogen in your combined contraception can affect your risk of developing breast cancer, but there isn't enough research to expand on this just yet or predict which combined pill brands have a higher or lower risk.

In 2023, new research[3] was published that also linked progestogen-only contraceptive methods to a slightly increased risk of breast cancer. The study revealed that there's a slightly increased risk of breast cancer in current or recent users of the progestogen-only pill, injection, implant or hormonal coil. But there was no significant difference between the types of progestogen-only methods and their effects on breast cancer.

Overall, people who use any method of hormonal contraception have a 20–30 per cent higher likelihood of developing breast cancer than non-users.[4] This seems scary, right? But this is relative risk, so let's put the risk into context and look at absolute numbers. If we imagine a city like Worcester (which has 100,000 people living in it) inhabited only by women aged sixteen to twenty-five, eight out of these 100,000 women (0.008 per cent) could develop breast cancer ten to fifteen years later if they were to use hormonal contraception for five years.[5] It's not a lot of extra cases. This risk does increase as women get older, but we know that breast cancer is a disease that generally affects older women. If Worcester is inhabited only by women aged thirty-five to thirty-nine who have used hormonal contraceptives for at least five years, there will be another 265 cases of breast cancer ten to fifteen years later (0.265 per cent).[6] It's important to stress that the risk of breast cancer in women during their reproductive years (i.e. users of contraception) is small and breast cancer is rare in women under thirty.[7]

There are over 56,000 cases of breast cancer each year in the UK. Of these, 8 per cent are caused by obesity and being overweight; 8 per cent are caused by drinking alcohol; and less than 1 per cent of cases are caused by oral contraceptives.[8]

**Causes of breast cancer each year in the UK**

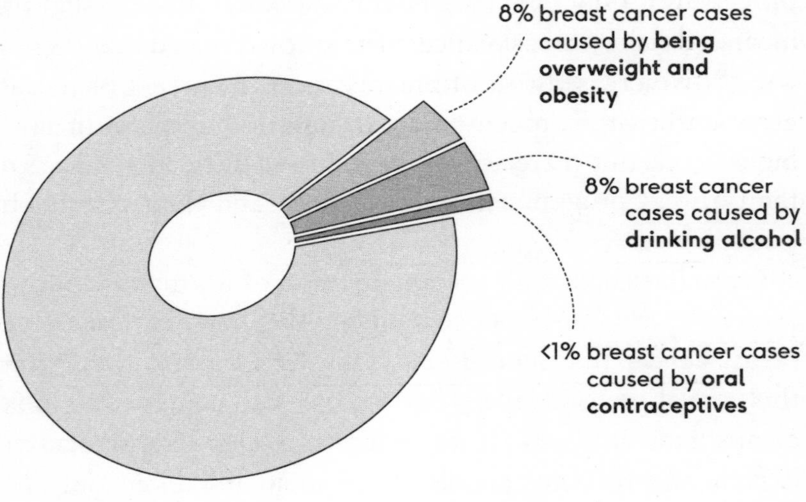


Based on data from Cancer Research UK. 56,822 new cases of breast cancer each year, 2017-2019 average, UK

So, your personal risk of developing breast cancer is also dependent on various other factors, aside from your contraception. As shown in the pie chart, factors like whether or not you drink alcohol, your weight and your genes all play a role, and the *most important* factor is your age. Another important point to keep in mind if you are weighing up the pros and cons of hormonal contraceptives is that the slightly elevated risk of breast cancer reduces once you stop using hormonal contraceptives, and ten years after you stop taking it, your risk will be back to normal.[9]

If you currently have breast cancer, you shouldn't use any form of hormonal contraception – but your doctor has probably already told you that. If you have a past history of breast cancer, you'd also need to consult your oncologist and cancer team before using hormonal contraception again. Everyone has BRCA genes, which protect us against breast and ovarian cancers. Some people have a faulty BRCA1 or BRCA2 gene, meaning this protective effect doesn't work as it should. If you know you carry a faulty BRCA gene (because you've had genetic testing), or you've been told you have a high risk of breast cancer by a breast or genetics doctor, due to significant family history, combined contraception is not advised, but UK guidance currently says that progestogen-only methods are considered safe to use.[10]

### *Cervical cancer*

So first off, and most importantly, hormonal contraceptives do not *cause* cervical cancer. They're not hormonally driven cancers and you can actually continue the pill, patch, vaginal ring, implant or injection while awaiting treatment for cervical cancer. The link between hormonal contraception and cervical cancer is most likely due to what we call 'confounding factors', i.e. other issues. For instance, if you use contraception, you're more likely to be having sex, so more likely to be exposed to human papillomavirus (HPV), a common virus spread through skin-to-skin and sexual contact, which causes almost all cervical cancers. But let's look at what the research shows.

One research article headline states that long-term use of

both the combined and the progestogen-only pill can increase your risk of cervical cancer by up to four times.[11] However, what you won't hear is that this research study *only* looked at women who were already infected with HPV, which is known to cause cervical cancer. So this four-times increased risk isn't fully representative of the whole female population.

Cancer Research UK states that for around 10 per cent of women in the UK who develop cervical cancer, this is linked to oral contraceptive use (*linked* but not *caused by*).[12] This risk increases the longer you're taking your contraception, with people who've been using hormonal contraception for five years or more having the greatest risk.[13] This might sound alarming, but around 3,200 women in the UK develop cervical cancer each year, so 10 per cent of these cases, only 320 (out of over thirty-four million women in the UK), each year are related to hormonal contraception. There is also evidence that the risk of cervical cancer diminishes once you stop taking hormonal contraception,[14] and to put it into perspective, less than 1 per cent of UK women develop cervical cancer during their lifetime.[15]

It's important to note that your risk of developing cervical cancer (whether you use hormonal contraceptives or not) is *extremely* low if you do not have human papillomavirus (HPV). You should also know that 99.8 per cent of cervical cancers are preventable,[16] which is why it's so important to attend your cervical screening appointments and get the HPV vaccination if you're eligible.

As an added extra, there is also evidence that users of the copper coil have reduced rates of both cervical cancer and endometrial cancer.[17]

### *Ovarian cancer*

Every time we ovulate, our ovaries are slightly damaged (talk about a design flaw). Damage to the ovaries over time can, in some cases, cause cancer. When we take oral hormonal contraception (which stops ovulation and prevents this damage from occurring), this can reduce the risk of developing ovarian cancer by 25–28 per cent.[18]

A huge study carried out in Denmark[19] found that this protective effect was more pronounced the longer a woman had been taking her contraception, and a meta-analysis (where lots of studies are pooled together) has shown that if you use oral contraceptives for ten years, your risk of ovarian cancer is reduced by a half, which is pretty mind blowing.[20] Other studies have found a benefit of decreased risk of ovarian cancer for up to thirty years after stopping hormonal contraception, but that this gradually reduces over time.[21]

There has been some research into the link between progestogen-only contraception and ovarian cancer, but the findings have been inconsistent. The Danish study previously mentioned didn't find any protective effects of progestogen-only contraception, though there are others that have. Using the hormonal coil has been associated with reduced cases of ovarian cancer,[22] as has the injection.[23] It's possible that inconsistencies in the research for progestogen-only contraception are because of the way certain progestogen-only contraceptives work, as not all of them always stop ovulation. It would be exciting to see further research being carried out in this area so that we can find out more.

### *Endometrial cancer*

This is a cancer that affects the lining of the uterus, and the news is good when it comes to contraception. Users of the combined pill have been found to have half the risk of developing endometrial cancer than those who have never used hormonal contraception.[24] And it's thought that in some cases, this protection could last up to twenty years after stopping contraception.[25]

Research into the effects of progestogen-only contraception on endometrial cancer risk is less common than other cancer research, but does suggest that these methods provide similar protection against the disease.[26] Research that looked at all oral contraceptive methods found a significant protective effect against endometrial cancer.[27] There is evidence that users of the hormonal and copper coil have reduced rates of both cervical cancer and endometrial cancer, up to 19 per cent.[28]

Using this amazing research, people who have periods less than every three months due to polycystic ovary syndrome are advised to use contraceptive options or progesterone tablets to keep the lining of the uterus thin to reduce their risk of cancerous changes over time.

### *Bowel cancer*

In even more promising news, a study[29] which followed 46,000 women to monitor the long-term impact of taking the combined contraceptive pill found that taking the pill for any length of time lowered the risk of bowel cancer. Researchers have also looked at all oral contraceptives together, rather than the progestogen-only pill alone, and have found a significant protective effect against bowel cancer (a reduction of 14–19 per cent).[30]

## Blood clots

Doctors use the terms venous thromboembolism (VTE), or more specifically deep vein thrombosis (DVT) or pulmonary embolism (PE) for what we commonly call blood clots, which can occur in the veins in the legs or lungs. Blood clotting is a vital process that prevents excessive bleeding – when we get a cut, the blood becomes sticky and clumps together to help stop us bleeding too much. But if clots form when and where they are not supposed to, the results can be dangerous. If a blood clot blocks a blood vessel it can prevent blood from reaching important organs and tissues or prevent oxygen from being transported from your lungs. In worst case scenarios, this can result in long-term damage, or death. Signs of a blood clot include throbbing or cramping pain in the leg or arm; swelling, redness and warmth in a leg or arm; sudden breathlessness, sharp chest pain (which may be worse when you breathe in) and coughing up blood. If you experience these, please immediately seek help.

Oestrogen can increase certain proteins in your blood that help it clot, known as clotting factors, and combined contraceptives containing both oestrogen and progestin have been shown to increase the risk of having a blood clot. Different contraceptive methods have different risks for blood clots and as with any medical decision, it's important to weigh up your personal risk. A contraceptive discussion with your GP, nurse or pharmacist should always cover your family and general medical history in order to assess this, taking into account if you or any first-degree relatives have had a blood clot before, especially at a young age, and any other risk factors for blood clots you may have, such as being a smoker or being overweight or obese. That said, the baseline risk of blood clots is so low that increasing it several times over will still result in a very small overall risk for most people.

So, what is the risk? Imagine 10,000 premenopausal women walking around right now who aren't using contraception. The number of them who will have a blood clot each year is around two.[31]

Women taking combined contraception have between two

and six times higher risk of developing blood clots.[32] This is relative risk so it sounds huge, but in reality there are still very few women who develop blood clots on the pill. Around nine to twelve women out of 10,000 will develop a clot while using a pill like Yasmin each year.[33] Of the small number of cases of blood clots that do occur in people using combined contraception, less than 1 per cent are fatal.[34] It's important to point out that if you have experienced a blood clot, the small risk to the general population doesn't matter . . . you've had a very scary experience, and this doesn't diminish that.

Blood clot risk is a complicated relationship between both the oestrogen and the progestogen parts of combined contraceptives. Different brands and types of combined contraception have different risks of blood clots. The table opposite summarises the increased risk with combined hormonal contraception based on progestogen type, including the actual number of women this risk corresponds to.

This is the reason why many people are first prescribed pill brands like Rigevidon, Microgynon or Ovranette, as these contain levonorgestrel and have the lowest blood clot risk. However, even if you are using a pill brand with a higher risk, such as Yasmin or Gedarel (perhaps because you've found the side effects are better, or it helps to manage conditions like acne or PCOS), the chance of getting a blood clot is *still* lower than if you are pregnant, or in the first six weeks after having a baby. Remember, we're always balancing risk against the risks of pregnancy, and contraception is designed to stop you from getting pregnant, so you're actually preventing a greater blood clot risk.

If you're taking a combined oral contraceptive pill your risk of blood clots is highest in the first three months after starting your contraception (if you've never taken it before).[35] In these cases, this may be because taking a combined hormonal

## Blood clot risk in users of combined contraception compared to baseline and risk in pregnancy or postpartum

| **Scenario** | **Estimated risk of developing a blood clot (VTE) in a year out of 10, 000 women*** |
|---|---|
| Not using contraception and not pregnant | 2 |
| Using combined contraception containing levonorgestrel, norethisterone or norgestimate e.g. Microgynon | 5 to 7 |
| Using combined contraception containing etonorgestrel or norelgestromin e.g. Evra patch and NuvaRing | 6 to 12 |
| Using combined contraception containing drospirenone, desogestrel or gestodene e.g Yasmin | 9 to 12 |
| | **Estimated risk of developing a blood clot (VTE) out of 10, 000 pregnant women**** |
| Pregnant or up to six weeks after delivery | 10 to 20 |

*European Medicines Agency. Press release: 'Benefits of combined hormonal contraceptives (CHCs) continue to outweigh risks', 2013.
**Royal College of Obstetricians and Gynaecologists, 'Reducing the risk of thrombosis and embolism during pregnancy and the puerperium' (Green-top Guideline No. 37a), 2015.

contraceptive can uncover any underlying or genetic clotting issues you might have. Your risk of blood clots could also increase if you stop taking combined hormonal contraception and then restart it again after more than four weeks.[36]

For most people, a small increase in the risk of blood clots isn't a concern. But if you or a family member have had a clot before, or your medical history predisposes you to blood clots, the overall risk becomes much higher, and your healthcare professional is trained to judge this. Progestogen-only methods are generally considered safe for you to use if combined contraceptives are not suitable for you due to increased blood clot risk.

---

**Q:** I have a relative who suffers from blood clots – does that mean the pill is a no-go for me?

**A:** Not necessarily. The UKMEC breaks down family history into family members who have had a blood clot before or after the age of forty-five, because having a blood clot at a younger age may in some cases point to a possible inherited condition. Doctors may also consider the circumstances under which your family member had the blood clot. However, this is a very individual discussion and decision, which may involve both your GP and a haematologist (blood clotting specialist) or a healthcare professional who really knows their stuff.

---

## Cardiovascular risk

For a small minority of users of combined contraception, the oestrogen part can cause raised blood pressure and increase the risk of heart attack and strokes. As with blood clot risk, the overall number of women using hormonal contraception who have a heart attack or stroke is exceptionally low and it's important to remember that pregnancy and the postpartum period inherently carry higher risks of these conditions than the use of hormonal contraceptives. The results of one large study from 2025 suggested that using the combined pill translates to one additional ischaemic stroke (caused by a blood clot in the arteries supplying the brain) per 4,760 women per year and one additional heart attack per 10,000 women per year.[37] The extremely low chance of having a stroke or heart attack seemed to increase with pills with higher amounts of oestrogen and with the patch and vaginal ring. Progestogen-only contraceptives showed little to no increased risk and the hormonal coil was not associated with an increased risk.[38] The other risk factors discussed below can increase the risk of heart and blood vessel problems:

- **Blood pressure** It's important if you're using combined methods, like the pill, patch or vaginal ring, that you have your blood pressure checked, as this is a risk factor for heart attacks or strokes. You need to have a recent blood pressure check before beginning your combined contraception and then every twelve months while you are taking it. This is also because combined contraception can cause an increase in blood pressure in some people.

If you see your healthcare professional in person, they will check your blood pressure using a machine with an inflatable cuff placed round your upper arm. This tightens then slowly releases before giving a blood pressure reading (some doctors will do this manually with an inflatable cuff and stethoscope). If you have a virtual consultation or order online, you can pop into a pharmacy for a quick check or buy your own blood pressure machine to use at home.

**Blood pressure readings**

Blood pressure readings come as two numbers, e.g. 120/80, and are measured in mmHg (millimetres of mercury). The top number is the systolic blood pressure, a measure of the force of pressure within your arteries when your heart muscle contracts. The bottom number is the diastolic blood pressure, a measure of the force of pressure within your arteries when your heart muscle is relaxed. Each heartbeat is your heart contracting and relaxing and it does this around sixty times a minute at rest.

Healthcare professionals won't prescribe new prescriptions or renew prescriptions for combined contraception without assessing your blood pressure reading. If you do have raised blood pressure, over 140/90 mmHg, you probably won't be prescribed combined hormonal contraceptives and may in fact require monitoring, follow-up and possible treatment to reduce your blood pressure. This is because raised blood pressure is a risk factor for heart and blood vessel disease and women with raised blood pressure who use combined contraception are therefore at further increased risk. If you are already using combined contraception then stopping it may improve your blood pressure. Raised blood pressure in pregnancy can cause significant complications, so ensuring you switch to another method to avoid unplanned pregnancy if you have raised blood pressure is important.

- **Smoking and vaping** Smoking increases your risk of cardiovascular disease and blood clots, so often we don't want to add more potential risks with combined hormonal contraception. The UKMEC looks at risk depending on

**Implant**
Used for 3–6 months   25 years old

★★★★★

**Nexplanon implant**

I love the implant. My doctor refused to renew my combination pill due to high blood pressure. At first I was really disappointed and angry because I had been really happy with that method and I was afraid that a new method would give me side effects. After five months, however, I haven't had any unwanted side effects whatsoever. The only change for me is that I don't get periods, but it's actually a bonus. During the first five months, I've had a tiny bit of spotting maybe twice and it only lasted a day, if that. I know everyone is different, but I would highly recommend the implant!

Shared on **thelowdown.com**

how many cigarettes you smoke, if and when you stopped and how old you are. This is used to stratify your risk and decide if you can have combined contraception. This might be a great time to start thinking about quitting. Check out places to get help in our Resources. Currently there is no guidance on the suitability of combined hormonal contraception in those who vape or use e-cigarettes due to the lack of any clear research evidence or data on safety. Until the studies show your risks of heart disease and blood clots are not increased with vaping and e-cigarettes, your doctor, nurse or pharmacist will consider the risks to be the same as smoking.[39]

- **Diabetes, high cholesterol and body mass index (BMI)** If you have diabetes (type 1 or 2), high cholesterol or your BMI is over 30, these can all increase your overall risk of having a heart attack or stroke. If you have several of these risk factors, your healthcare professional will assess these alongside your age to decide if combined contraception is too risky for you. A note on BMI: this number, generated from your height and weight, is a really useful tool to assess a large number of people's overall health related to their weight. But we have to remember that some people (e.g. athletes) can have a high BMI and still be incredibly healthy due to their muscle mass. It's not a perfect score, and doesn't determine your overall health as an individual, as other indicators, such as waist circumference and body fat percentage, may give a more accurate picture. But BMI has been used in most medical research studies as a marker of health, so this is why healthcare professionals use it in their guidance.
- **Migraine** Migraine is a really common reason to be denied the combined pill. Especially migraine with aura. Aura is a term used to describe any sort of neurological disturbance which can appear before the headache or other symptoms of a migraine. Often visual, these include flashing lights, coloured spots or zigzag lines in the field of vision. This can be extremely frightening the first time it happens but typically subsides within an hour. Other neurological symptoms such as weakness on one side, dizziness or vertigo can occur too. These symptoms can be difficult to differentiate from emergencies like having a stroke, so will often require an urgent medical assessment when they first happen.

If you have migraine with aura and use the combined pill, the evidence is limited but suggests you may have up to a six times higher risk of having a stroke compared to women who don't use the combined pill.[40] This statement refers to relative risk and it's important to remember that the chance of having a stroke in women of reproductive age is actually very low. However, strokes can be completely debilitating and disabling, so for young women, the additional risk just isn't worth it. If you have migraines *without* aura, the rules are slightly different. You can start the combined pill if you have plain old migraines, and continue it if they don't get worse. However, if you start to get migraines for the first time when you start taking the pill, or your existing migraines worsen, it's advised that you choose another method.[41]

## Fertility

There is a really common myth that contraception affects your fertility, or ability to conceive and have a child in the future. Women tend to worry about this, either when they're thinking about it for the future or when they've stopped their contraceptive and are desperate to be pregnant. Let's address that head-on with what research says to ease your mind.

- **Pills, patches, rings, implants and coils** For nearly all contraceptive methods, fertility returns very quickly as soon as you've stopped using it. The majority of women will ovulate within a month of stopping the pill, and there is no evidence to suggest the use of these contraceptives has any long-term impact on fertility, including if you've been taking the combined pill back to back.[42] Some may be concerned about the length of time they've been on the pill, but this, too, has no impact according to the research. In fact, pregnancy rates in the first one to two years after stopping the pill are the same as for couples who have only used condoms or no contraception at all.[43]

It is important to remember when you stop using your

method, your fertility will return to whatever is normal for you. There may be underlying factors that *aren't* related to your contraception which still affect your fertility, such as your age, or conditions like PCOS and endometriosis. If you have a male partner, their fertility could also be a factor.

- **The injection** This is the only form of hormonal contraception that can impact your fertility for a short time after stopping, and research has shown that it takes longer for couples to get pregnant after using the injection than any other method.[44] This impact isn't permanent and we'll cover it more in Chapter 9. Worrying about your cycle and fertility returning after stopping the injection can be super stressful, so some users try to plan ahead and think about switching to a different option in the one to two years before they're considering starting a family.

### The risks associated with procedures and devices

- **Coil insertion** With any procedure, there are always risks. The main risks are pain, infection and bleeding. For coil insertion, we've discussed how to manage pain in Chapter 3. Other risks you should know about are listed here.

  - There is a very small chance of infection after a coil is fitted, which increases in the first three weeks after it's inserted.[45] You can usually tell as your vaginal discharge may become green or smell bad, and you can get a fever or heavy/abnormal bleeding. If this happens, please see a healthcare professional who can prescribe antibiotics. In most cases, these work well and the coil doesn't need to be removed.
  - Expulsion (the term used to describe the coil essentially falling out) happens for one in every twenty coil

fittings, most commonly in the first three months.[46] There can also be a partial expulsion where the coil moves down from its ideal place in the uterus and can sit lower in the cervix. This can often cause pain, especially during sex, and you may be able to feel the coil during sex or have abnormal bleeding. Factors which make expulsion more likely include if you're a teenager, have very heavy periods or fibroids, or use a menstrual cup.[47] Remember to avoid sex or use an alternative form of contraception if you can't feel your threads or notice your coil in the toilet!

- Perforation is probably the scariest risk of coil insertion, and this is where the coil moves and can put a small hole in the wall of the uterus. Thankfully this is rare, only occurring in one to two in 1,000 coil fittings (0.1–0.2 per cent).[48] Usually these are diagnosed via an ultrasound or pelvic X-ray if you complain of having lower tummy pain or unusual bleeding, especially if the threads can't be seen or felt. The coil is then removed, sometimes using a camera in an outpatient clinic or, rarely, with keyhole surgery. Breastfeeding can also increase the chances of a perforation, so some practitioners may advise trying to avoid breastfeeding for three to eight hours after insertion, but there is no research to support recommending this.[49]
- Ovarian cysts could be classed as a risk or a side effect of coils. There has been a reported increase in the risk of ovarian cysts with women who use hormonal coils, and this may be related to the size (and dose of progestogen) of the coils. However, this increased risk doesn't seem to be clinically significant, as the vast majority of cysts do not cause symptoms and 80–90 per cent resolve by themselves within three months.[50]

Importantly, if you have had or currently have an ovarian cyst, or suffer from PCOS, you can have a hormonal coil if this is your preferred choice.

- If you were to get pregnant with a copper or hormonal coil in place, a higher *proportion* of these pregnancies are ectopic (where the pregnancy is not in the uterus but elsewhere, commonly the fallopian tube), than if you were to fall pregnant naturally without a coil in place. However, the effectiveness of the coils is so high, that the risk of ectopic pregnancy with a coil is still much lower than using no contraception at all. The research is undecided as to whether the hormonal or copper coils have a higher ectopic pregnancy risk, but there is some very limited research that suggests the proportion of ectopic pregnancies may be higher in people who fall pregnant with lower dose hormonal coils (like the Jaydess).[51]

• **Implant insertion** Implant insertion is exceptionally safe with pain (one in twenty), bruising or bleeding (one in fifty) being the main complications.[52] There are some less common things to be aware of, however:

- Implant migration. Just like birds in winter, implants have been known to move around. If correctly inserted, implants can move, but only by around 2 cm in total. There have been a handful of cases reported where the implant has moved elsewhere. In eleven cases the implant moved to the armpit, and in one case to the shoulder.[53] Most bizarrely, some implants have ended up in the veins in the lungs, but this is so vanishingly rare, it happens for only one in every 1.3 million implants sold according to the manufacturer.[54]

- Nerve or muscle damage caused by implant insertion are typically explained as theoretical risks, but there's literally no decent research to back up whether this has happened and how often.

• **Sterilisation** Female sterilisation is a surgical procedure, so it comes with risks of pain, bleeding and infection. You also need to consider the risks of the anaesthetic used, which will be assessed by an anaesthetist or pre-operative nurse before your procedure. Rarely, during the procedure, there may be damage to the bladder, bowel or blood vessels which requires a larger operation to fix. You will need to sign a consent form prior to sterilisation to confirm that these risks have been discussed and you understand them all.

• **Vasectomy** Vasectomies are carried out under local anaesthetic, which has very few risks. The infection risk is 0.2–1.5 per cent.[55] One in 300 men may develop scrotal pain after a vasectomy.[56] We can reassure men, however, that sexual function is not affected.[57]

### Other risks to be aware of

• **The injection and bone density** Bone mass density is the marker of how strong your bones are. Generally, if it is lower, you're more likely to break a bone. Bone mass declines as we get older, especially after menopause, and is also affected by your family history, BMI and if you smoke or drink alcohol. The contraceptive injection is associated with a loss of bone density. However, the difference in bone mass density between women who used the Depo-Provera injection and those who used non-hormonal methods wasn't significant until they'd been using the injection for thirteen to fifteen years.[58] It's been noted that the loss of bone density is quickest in the first year of use,[59] but then the rate tapers off with time.[60] Thankfully, this is only temporary and bone mass recovers to baseline after the injection has been stopped.[61]

Practically, this means that certain injection users need to be aware of this risk. Especially those under the age of eighteen (when bones are still growing) or nearing menopause. The guidance recommends that the risk of bone density loss is discussed every two years while using the injection, and anyone under the age of eighteen should be properly counselled on other options. And when you hit fifty years old, you should switch to an alternative option.[62]

• **Meningioma and progestogens** Meningioma is an uncommon and usually benign tumour. It's not cancerous but can cause other problems by pressing on brain tissue, so may require surgery. It's very rare under the age of thirty-five; however, the risk increases as you get older, with most people diagnosed over the age of sixty-five.[63]

Studies have found a small increased risk of meningioma requiring surgery in people who had used the synthetic progestogens cyproterone acetate (which is in the combined pill Dianette) and nomegestrol acetate (at higher doses than in the combined pill Zoely).[64] People with meningioma should not use these contraceptives.[65] Another study has also suggested a link between the risk of meningioma and the prolonged use of medroxyprogesterone acetate, the progestogen in the contraceptive injections Depo Provera and Sayana Press.[66] The FSRH have suggested that clinicians should include this new info in conversations around risk and benefits of contraception with patients and they will be monitoring the evidence around progestogen use and risk of meningioma. But for now, this is just something to be aware of.[67]

## Following the evidence about risk

This chapter may have been a *lot* to take in – understanding risk is not an easy concept. When it comes to any part of your health, getting the facts that allow you to make a decision that feels right to you is essential. We need to be cautious too about where we get this info to ensure it's from a trustworthy source that is based on evidence, to save you from social media doomscrolling. Medical advice or research should usually always have a publication date (so that you can see how up-to-date it is), and if references are used they should be cited from credible sources.

You might have noticed in recent years a rise in self-proclaimed 'experts' on social media giving medical advice. This content often feels unsettling, focusing on the health risks and damaging side effects of just about everything. Plenty of these rants are about contraception too, often based on nonsense – given by people with zero medical expertise, some of whom deliberately want to mislead. These articles and videos can be so convincing, cleverly playing on our worries around side effects and illness, leaving many people fearful of all hormonal contraception.

Women's health conditions and contraception are under-researched and overlooked areas, so it's no surprise that there's a hotbed of misinformation. Contraception myths often stem from a misunderstanding of how the science works, scaremongering or simply drawing on outdated or refuted science and guidance. We often avoid asking healthcare professionals questions about risk because we've had unhelpful experiences in the past, are afraid of coming across as idiotic, or just can't get an appointment to see them in the first place. So, we look to the people around us for facts and advice, or to Dr Google, which can churn up a whole sea of misinformation if we don't look in the right places. Be mindful of where you get your intel – we have included some of our go-to sources for evidence-based medical info in the Resources section.

It can be heartbreaking and scary to see a video pop up of someone telling their personal horror story with contraception, in which they had an extreme reaction resulting in hospitalisation. These cases often get picked up by the media, adding to the panic. We don't want to diminish these women's awful experiences with contraception, far from it. Our core principle is to give everyone a voice to share their experience with contraception to push for much-needed research. But it is important to remember that everyone is different, and the likelihood of these things happening to you, the person reading this book, who is now armed with all the information you need to know about what contraception is likely to be suited to you, is small.

# 7

# Switching and stopping contraception

Most of us have a reproductive lifespan of around thirty years. During this time, our needs will naturally evolve, and the contraception that suited us decades ago may no longer serve us so well now. In fact, the average person stops, starts or changes their contraceptive method up to ten times in their lifetime.[1]

Research shows that around three-quarters of people stopping or switching their contraception list side effects as a reason,[2] and Lowdown data backs this up by showing that the top reason people stopped using the method they've reviewed on our site is that they didn't like the side effects.[3] This leads to many of us questioning whether the benefits are worth it and whether switching – or stopping altogether – might be the best solution.

Have you ever taken a break from a method and found you feel different when you return to it? Many women tell us their side effects change when they return to a contraceptive method again after a long break, like after having a baby. We'll bust some common myths – for example, *could* your contraceptive be impacting your personality? – and dive into what you need to know about how to stop, take a break and/or safely switch your brand or method. Whether you're facing unwanted side effects from your current contraceptive or it's no longer suiting your lifestyle, we've already established in this book that there are, fortunately, other options out there. So consider this chapter a handy toolkit to help you prepare for the changes that could arise in the first few months of stopping or switching your contraception.

## Switching from a method due to health risks

Most of us will be advised by our doctor that it is safe to continue using hormonal contraception as long as we're feeling well and our medical history doesn't change. However, a small minority of people may be advised that the potential risks of certain methods could outweigh the benefits. This might be due to a number of reasons, such as being over the age of fifty, when combined hormonal contraception and the injection are not recommended (as the associated risks increase with age). Similarly, if you've had any changes to your medical history, like you discover you have raised blood pressure, experience migraine with aura, gain weight so your BMI is over 35, continue to smoke over the age of thirty-five or discover you are a faulty BRCA gene carrier, your healthcare professional will no longer be able to safely offer you combined hormonal methods.[4] You should have an annual contraception review to screen for any changes like this in your medical history and in these cases, your healthcare professional should discuss alternative contraceptives with you. If any new medical symptoms or medications crop up before your next review, seek advice in case they affect the safety of your current contraceptive.

We looked at the main risks associated with taking

hormonal contraception in Chapter 6, so head back for a reminder, if needed.

**Combined pill**
Used for 18 months to 3 years  40 years old

★★★★☆

**Microgynon 30 pill**

I was very happy using Microgynon as it didn't seem to have many side effects at all. However, while using it I was diagnosed with high blood pressure and since stopping the pill my blood pressure has returned to normal levels.

Shared on **thelowdown.com**

## Contraception and the three-month rule

If you've started a new contraceptive, you'll probably have been warned about the potential side effects that might crop up. Your healthcare professional is also likely to give a timeframe in which you can hope to see these ease up, which is where the three-month rule comes in. This is based on the idea that, for some people, it can take around this time for your body to adjust to the hormones (or the copper coil). But is three really the magic number when it comes to figuring out if the contraceptive you've started is right for you? Well, research shows that side effects (in particular bloating, nausea and breast tenderness) usually do subside in the first three months.[5] For this reason, provided the side effects are manageable, your best bet may be to wait it out. That can be easier said than done – three months is a long time to feel off your A-game. And as we mentioned in Chapter 5 on side effects, it could take even longer for some side effects, like bleeding, to settle down.

**Implant**
Used for 12–18 months · 28 years old

★★★☆☆

**Nexplanon implant**

It was my first time on contraception, so I was afraid to forget the pill and had the feeling that the implant had fewer hormones in it. My mood was very fluctuating for the first four to six months but then settled. My period was much lighter at the beginning and not painful for the first few months, then actually got irregular after seven to eight months (only a few days, then nothing for two weeks, then three weeks long period . . .). The insertion of the implant was very easy and not too painful – I've been able to feel it since the beginning.

Shared on **thelowdown.com**

While most people find their body adjusts during this timeframe, some will not. Talking to your healthcare professional to find ways to manage side effects is always an option. Make sure you're clued up on any serious symptoms that may require immediate medical attention (by reading your patient information leaflet carefully) rather than waiting it out, though.

**Q:** Are there any side effects which won't settle after three months?

**A:** The majority of side effects will improve within three to six months if you can manage them until then. The most common exception to this rule seen in clinical practice is bleeding with the implant. The bleeding pattern with the implant is unpredictable, and it can change at any time. In fact, one study found that 25 per cent of users had no bleeding at all in the first year, but this reduced to 12 per cent in the third year of use,[6] meaning some women's bleeds started again!

## How to safely switch your contraception

So, you've made a decision and you're about to start your new contraceptive or switch to a different option. We wish switching could always be simple, but as with everything contraception-related, it can be a little complicated. Switching between contraceptive methods can be a risky time for pregnancy, if not done correctly. We've summarised guidance from the FSRH on how to switch your contraception safely[7] on our website (see Resources), but remember this guidance should never be used as a substitute for individual medical advice and you should always speak to your doctor, nurse or pharmacist before switching methods if you have any questions or concerns. If in doubt, consider using additional contraception, such as condoms, until you are certain your new method has started working.

Do you ***need*** to take a break from hormonal contraception?

So, there are loads of reasons why you might want to take a breather from your contraception, but the question is: do you *need* to?

Actually, there is no medical reason for most of us to have a long-term break from our contraceptive. Some people understandably worry about the effects synthetic hormones might have on them. There can be a concern that they'll build up in the body or that having these additional hormones in the bloodstream means organs need to work harder. Reassuringly, though, that's not the case. Most methods of hormonal contraception work to stop ovulation, preventing fertilisation of an egg and, as a result, pregnancy. The hormones in contraception that make this happen essentially pause the menstrual cycle. So, there's no build-up of hormones or excess stress put on the body that requires our organs to compensate. Similarly, you don't need to worry about a build up of blood with nowhere to go – hormonal contraceptives thin the uterus lining so there is no blood that needs to come out.

- **Blood clot risk** As we looked at in Chapter 6, there is a small risk of blood clots associated with combined hormonal contraception. Something to be mindful of, too, is that stopping and restarting combined hormonal contraception can increase this risk. The risk of blood clots with combined oral contraceptives is highest when you start the method for the very first time.[8] This may be because taking a combined hormonal contraceptive can uncover any blood clotting issues you might naturally have. Research has shown that your risk of blood clots could also be higher if you stop taking combined contraception for four weeks or more, and then restart it again.[9]

## When do you no longer need contraception because you can't get pregnant any more?

The day you stop needing to use contraception is without a doubt a milestone. Some people find it's one less thing to worry about as you get older, while others might feel a sense of loss. You may have opted to have a permanent contraceptive procedure or needed to have a hysterectomy to treat another condition. Whether it was your choice or not, it's normal to have mixed feelings about it.

• **Age** The following age-related advice is only relevant if you're not using hormonal contraception (which, as you now know, can stop periods). You no longer need contraception:[10]

- Two years after your last period if you're between the ages of forty and fifty.
- One year after your last period if you're over the age of fifty.

From the age of fifty-five, there is no longer any need for contraception because the risk of spontaneous pregnancy is so low, even if you're still having periods.[11] We get asked about using contraception in your forties and fifties so often, and whether you need to change how you use it. So we've dedicated a chapter to contraception in perimenopause and menopause later on.

• **Male and female sterilisation** Your partner getting a vasectomy can herald a new era of unprotected sex. Don't throw out your contraception immediately, though, as a vasectomy should only be relied upon after semen testing shows there are no more sperm in the ejaculate (see page 99). It usually takes around twelve weeks to get the all-clear from a doctor.[12] Getting your tubes tied (i.e. female sterilisation, page 99) is another highly effective method of preventing pregnancy. Remember, though, that barrier methods like condoms may still be needed to protect against STIs.

• **After a hysterectomy** Surgical procedures such as a hysterectomy will mean it is impossible to become pregnant, and so contraception is no longer necessary. You may choose to have a hysterectomy to help treat adenomyosis symptoms or manage heavy periods and pain from fibroids, or it might be necessary as part of cancer treatment.

## How to stop taking hormonal contraception

So, you've decided to break up with hormonal contraception. But how do you actually stop? Different hormonal methods require different actions (or inaction) to stop using it. Some types allow you to easily stop by yourself while others require a healthcare professional to be involved. One thing that is common across all methods, though, is, unlike some other medication, you do not need to gradually wean yourself off hormonal contraception. This myth pops up now and again (often from dodgy online sources) but it's completely untrue. You also don't need to have blood tests or take a load of supplements to 'support yourself coming off the pill'.

• **Oral contraception** Whatever the type or brand of pill, you can simply just stop taking it. When you do, you're no longer protected from pregnancy.

• **Patch and vaginal ring** Similar to the pill, simply remove the patch or ring and do not replace. After removing, you're no longer protected from pregnancy.

• **Important note for combined pills, patch and ring or the drospirenone-based progestogen-only pill (like Slynd)** If you do not wish to become pregnant and have been having unprotected sex, make sure you have taken the method consistently and correctly for seven days before stopping and consider switching to an alternative method. This may mean restarting your pill after a scheduled pill-free break if you have had unprotected sex in this time.[13]

- **Injection** The Depo-Provera and Sayana Press injections are given every thirteen weeks, and can't be removed or stopped once given. So if you'd like to stop, just wait for the effects to wear off and do not get the next injection after thirteen weeks.
- **Hormonal and non-hormonal coil or implant** You'll need to schedule an appointment with a healthcare professional to have these removed. Do not try to remove your own coil, however tempted you may be! Yes, it seems easy for clinicians to remove, but trust us, it takes some skill and you don't want to damage the cervix and get a load of blood all over your sofa cushions. Please leave it to the professionals. For these methods, you should be advised to abstain from sex or use condoms for seven days before having them removed if you want to avoid pregnancy. This is because sperm can stay alive for several days after unprotected sex and if you ovulate soon after the coil is removed there is potential for the sperm to meet and fertilise an egg.

For all methods, if you want to avoid pregnancy, you'll need to use another form of contraception straight away. This can be a bit of an adjustment if you've been exclusively using hormonal contraception for a while. Think about these practicalities in advance and get organised – this may simply mean stocking up on condoms or making an appointment with your GP, nurse or pharmacist to discuss other options.

On page 80, we look at non-hormonal short and long-term options that will help protect you effectively from pregnancy. You can always come back to the switching contraception guide we've linked to in Resources to make sure you're safely switching contraception during the transition.

## What to watch out for when you quit hormonal contraception

If you can't remember what it feels like without synthetic hormones in your system, you're in good company. Lots of people tell us they're trying to rediscover who they 'really are' by taking a break from hormonal contraception. So, where do the side effects of synthetic hormones end and our real personalities begin? If you've been taking hormonal contraception for many years, even before you were an adult, you might be intrigued to find out whether you'll feel different once you stop using it.

It's important to say that lots of people quit their hormonal method and don't feel much, if any, difference. They get on with life, often pleasantly surprised that there are few changes (aside from their period returning or maybe becoming slightly heavier). For a minority, though, it's a massive shift, where they feel their personality has been transformed to their 'true' self after synthetic hormones. Some report a positive impact on their mood, however, for others, it can feel like they're unravelling as they start to suffer from more negative mood symptoms which may be related to PMS or PMDD. On pages 216–217 we summarise some findings from our users who told us about changes to their moods and emotions after stopping their contraceptives.

---

**Q:** I've heard that my sexual preferences may change when I come off hormonal contraception, even the people I'm attracted to – is this true?

**A:** Anecdotally, we've heard from people who felt like their contraception changed their sexuality, with the most extreme stories including people suddenly being attracted to another gender after coming off it or on starting a new method. We ran a small Instagram poll asking if anyone felt like the pill had changed their sexuality, and 1,362 people responded. Twenty-two per cent said yes, a little; 5 per cent said yes, completely; and 73 per cent said no.[14] Sexuality refers to a person's sexual feelings, attraction to others and how they express those feelings and preferences, and includes sexual orientation, behaviour and identity. Lots of external factors can contribute to a shift in sexuality, which is totally normal. Evolutionary psychologist Sarah E. Hill suggests that it could be plausible that hormonal contraception can affect sexuality, as sex hormones can be involved in sexual attraction. She argues that for some people, the hormonal changes from hormonal contraception could shift their preferences in ways that are more noticeable than others.[15] When it comes to sexual attraction, there's actually, rather surprisingly, quite a bit of psychological research on the subject. But this has all focused on how cis women are attracted to typical cis male features and if this could be affected by contraceptives (guess who's been funding this research . . .). In the early twenty-first century, studies hypothesised that hormonal variations throughout a female menstrual cycle changed how attracted they were to men – with women being attracted to more masculine features when they were ovulating and at peak fertility. The authors of these studies were concerned that using the pill could alter these responses.[16] However, since then, three much larger studies have found no evidence that the pill affects who women are attracted to or the quality of their long-term relationships.[17] And we need to be reminded that sexuality and relationships are so complex that it's unlikely one factor (like your contraception) will impact your decision to start, or indeed leave, a relationship.

## How Lowdown reviewers report that contraception changed their mood after they stopped using it

Reviewers were asked: *After* you stopped using this contraception, did you notice any changes to your moods and emotions? Reviewers could select one option.

| | Very positively | Somewhat positively |
|---|---|---|
| **Combined pill** | 14% | 15% |
| **Progestogen-only pill** | 14% | 14% |
| **Hormonal coil (IUS)** | 11% | 10% |
| **Implant** | 11% | 14% |
| **Copper coil (IUD)** | 7% | 8% |
| **Injection** | 15% | 22% |
| **Patch** | 18% | 21% |
| **Vaginal ring** | 40% | 0% |

| Neutral / no change | Somewhat negatively | Very negatively | I don't know / can't tell |
|---|---|---|---|
| 16% | 23% | 26% | 6% |
| 14% | 22% | 26% | 10% |
| 26% | 18% | 23% | 12% |
| 12% | 22% | 32% | 9% |
| 51% | 15% | 12% | 7% |
| 20% | 20% | 18% | 5% |
| 25% | 14% | 14% | 8% |
| 40% | 20% | 0% | 0% |

Analysis of The Lowdown contraception review data July 2024. 688 combined pill reviews, 304 progestogen-only pill reviews, 156 hormonal coil (IUS) reviews, 202 implant reviews, 137 copper coil (IUD) reviews, 115 injection reviews, 28 patch reviews, 5 vaginal ring reviews.

## When will your period come back?

When periods return after stopping hormonal contraception can vary from person to person, and the method you've been using can impact this too. On average, the injection generally takes the longest for periods to return to normal. But most contraception users find their normal cycle returns in the first few months after they stop using their method. The first bleed you have after stopping combined methods is actually a withdrawal bleed rather than a period. This is a result of the synthetic hormones leaving your body and it may last up to seven days. Usually, your second bleed is your period, as a result of the return of your menstrual cycle. The table on pages 220–221 shows how long Lowdown reviewers reported it took for their periods to return to what was normal for them. This doesn't factor in whether reviewers had other problems impacting the return of their periods. We discuss this more in 'What is "masking"?'

---

**Q:** Can I still get pregnant if my periods haven't returned?

**A:** Yes, you can! Be mindful that for most people their fertility will return straight away, and that you are most fertile around ovulation, which occurs around two weeks before you have a period, meaning it's possible to get pregnant before your first period.

If you've been using contraceptives for years, you may not even remember much about your cycle, especially if you started using contraception as a teenager. If you did have a monthly bleed on combined hormonal contraception, you'll also know from Chapter 2 that it was a withdrawal bleed rather than a true period. Though you likely thought about it in much the same way as a period (bleeding to manage, period products to use, leakage mishaps to launder). Similarly, if your contraception has put a stop to your periods, either through continuous use or as a side effect, then get ready to be reacquainted with your monthly bleed. It can take a while for things to return to what's normal for you, and you might find your cycle is a completely new 'normal' to what it was before. If after three to six months your cycle is longer than thirty-five days or you're bleeding in between your periods, see your GP.

---

## What is 'masking'?

While your hormonal contraception was doing its thing, it could have also been effectively managing or treating an underlying medical condition and/or unwanted symptoms from your menstrual cycle. While this is usually a great benefit, we've heard from people who worry that their contraception may just be 'masking' their symptoms. As we've seen, many people start taking hormonal contraception to treat issues with their cycle or to manage gynaecological conditions. When they stop taking hormones, these problems may still be lurking, as there is no cure for conditions like polycystic ovary syndrome (PCOS) or endometriosis. In fact, some conditions only become apparent to people once they come off hormonal contraceptives or are trying to get pregnant.

In Chapter 4, we looked at some of the most common conditions that are often managed with hormonal contraception: bleeding issues like heavy or painful periods, fibroids, endometriosis, adenomyosis, acne, PCOS, menstrual migraines and PMS or PMDD. For some people, contraception used in this way can work wonders to manage their debilitating symptoms. So it makes sense that coming off contraception may cause a

## How long Lowdown reviewers report that it took their menstrual cycle to return to normal after they stopped using contraception

Reviewers were asked: How long did it take for your period cycle to return to normal after you stopped using this method of contraception? We know everyone's version of 'normal' is different. Please let us know how long it takes for your periods to get into their normal rhythm. Reviewers could select one option.

| | **1-2 months** | **3-6 months** | **6-12 months** |
|---|---|---|---|
| **Combined pill** | 43% | 13% | 5% |
| **Progestogen-only pill** | 44% | 14% | 4% |
| **Implant** | 52% | 14% | 4% |
| **Hormonal coil (IUS)** | 44% | 19% | 5% |
| **Copper coil (IUD)** | 59% | 7% | 1% |
| **Injection** | 9% | 16% | 20% |
| **Patch** | 54% | 11% | 0% |
| **Vaginal ring** | 40% | 0% | 20% |

| 12–18 months | 18 months – 3 years | 3+ years | Don't know / can't tell |
|---|---|---|---|
| 2% | 1% | 0% | 36% |
| 1% | 0% | 0% | 37% |
| 1% | 0% | 0% | 29% |
| 0% | 1% | 1% | 30% |
| 0% | 1% | 0% | 32% |
| 11% | 4% | 0% | 40% |
| 0% | 3% | 0% | 32% |
| 0% | 0% | 20% | 20% |

Analysis of The Lowdown contraception review data July 2024. 698 combined pill reviews, 310 progestogen-only pill reviews, 203 implant reviews, 156 hormonal coil (IUS) reviews, 137 copper coil (IUD) reviews, 114 injection reviews, 28 patch reviews, 5 vaginal ring reviews.

return of these problems. This is not a given, though, and some people find they feel better. Hormonal contraceptives can also mask (or we could say … treat) symptoms of perimenopause, which we'll be looking at more closely in Chapter 11.

Fortunately, there are alternative treatments to manage a return of symptoms when you no longer get the benefits from your contraception (we touched on some of these in Chapter 4). Whatever your reasons for coming off hormonal contraception, it's a good idea to discuss this with a healthcare professional in advance of stopping. They will help you make a plan for managing a potential return of symptoms, and if you want to switch to another method, you can discuss your options together.

# 8

# Plan B – and what to do if Plan B fails

• **Content warning** This chapter contains descriptions of what happens during an abortion.

Split condoms, missed pills or no contraception at all – accidents happen, and it's important to know that, firstly, that's OK. Knowing the ins and outs of emergency contraception and how it works will help you not to panic if the time comes when you need to use it. If you do find yourself unexpectedly pregnant, we've laid out your options in this chapter for what to do next.

Around half of women who accidentally fall pregnant are using contraception (but mostly using it incorrectly or inconsistently).[1] Even if you are vigilant about using your contraception by the book, on rare occasions pregnancy can still occur. It can feel overwhelming and scary, but in the UK there are organisations in place to help you navigate the practical and emotional side of unplanned pregnancy (see Resources). Accidental pregnancy is really common, even among the super-conscientious, but it can sometimes feel like you're the only person you know that this has happened to. The reality is that it's probably happened, or will happen, to someone you know at some point in their life too. Whether you choose to disclose it to people around you or not is completely up to you, but just know that you're not alone.

Around the world, there are different laws and practices around accessing emergency contraception and abortion. The info in this chapter relates to the UK, so organisations, services and your options may vary if you are elsewhere.

## Emergency contraception

If you've had unprotected sex and don't want to become pregnant, using emergency contraception is your best bet. 'Unprotected' sex means any time you have sex and don't use contraception, or it's not used correctly, or has failed. This could include things like a condom breaking, not taking a pill or something happening to make your pill less effective (see Chapter 2, page 35). There are two types of emergency contraceptives: oral emergency contraception (most commonly known as the morning after pill) and the copper coil (IUD). Timing is everything with emergency contraception – generally, the sooner you use it, the higher the chances of it working.

If you're taking oral contraceptives (aka the pill), and are late taking a pill or have missed one altogether, use The Lowdown's online missed pill calculator (see Resources section for a direct link). This is the first online tool of its kind. We created it because time and time again women were coming to us asking for advice on what to do if they had missed a pill. Huge patient information leaflets with minuscule writing and confusing instructions just weren't cutting it. Our calculator takes all the guesswork out of it, asking a series of simple questions to give you an answer based on a traffic-light system with instructions on what to do next. Green means no need for emergency contraception, amber means you're potentially at risk of pregnancy, and red means you're at high risk. If in doubt, always contact a healthcare professional for advice.

## The copper coil

Not many people know this, but the copper coil (also called IUD) is *the* most effective form of emergency contraception and should be offered to everyone needing emergency contraception. Fewer than 0.1 per cent of people become pregnant after having the copper coil fitted as emergency contraception, and it can be used within five days of unprotected sex or up to five days after your earliest possible ovulation date for that cycle. So there's often more leeway than the emergency contraceptive pill. The copper IUD has toxic effects on the sperm and egg which prevents them meeting and the egg being fertilised. It also affects the lining of the uterus so that if an egg was fertilised, it won't be able to implant in the uterus lining at all. This is a non-hormonal method, with the added benefit of being able to remain in place as a long-term contraceptive (it can last five to ten years depending on the brand, though it can be removed any time before then if you'd like). Unlike the emergency contraceptive pill, your body mass index (BMI) does not impact the effectiveness of the copper coil. However, it isn't suitable for everyone, so a healthcare professional can help you assess whether it's a viable option for you. Your GP or local sexual health service will have a protocol to make sure you get seen and sorted with an emergency IUD quickly after unprotected sex. See page 66 for more info about coil fitting.

**Q:** I want to use the copper coil as emergency contraception but I don't want to keep it in long term. Can it be removed quickly and easily once it has acted as emergency contraception?

**A:** Absolutely. If you don't want to keep the copper coil in long term, you can have it removed after you are sure you are not pregnant. You should do a pregnancy test three weeks after unprotected sex to check. In the very rare case that it's positive, speak to a healthcare professional and tell them you have a copper coil in place.

### Emergency contraceptive pills aka 'the morning after pill'

Emergency contraceptive pills can be used to prevent pregnancy in the hours or days after unprotected sex, not just the 'morning after' as their commonly used name suggests. But the window of time you have to take it after unprotected sex will depend on the type of pill you take. In the UK, there are two different types of emergency contraceptive pills available. We surveyed 1,068 people, and a huge 73 per cent didn't know that there were two different types.[2] But it's important to know this, because the type and dose that will work best for you will depend on things like how long ago you had unprotected sex, your BMI and whether you use hormonal contraception. Here's a super quick overview of them:

- The levonorgestrel pill (brand names include Levonelle, Ezinelle, LoviOne or Plan B) contains the synthetic hormone levonorgestrel, a type of

progestogen, and can be taken up to seventy-two hours (three days) after unprotected sex. Levonorgestrel is the same type of progestogen used in pills like Microgynon, just in a larger dose. Because it's been around for years, and is in so many pill brands, we know it's super safe to use.
- The other type of emergency contraceptive pill, which contains a hormone modulator called ulipristal acetate (brand name ellaOne), can be taken up to 120 hours (five days) after unprotected sex and is more effective than levonorgestrel.

*How do emergency contraceptive pills work?*

Another thing a lot of people don't know is that the primary function of the emergency contraceptive pill is to delay ovulation so that the sperm from unprotected sex are no longer around by the time an egg is released. Without fertilisation between a sperm and an egg, pregnancy can't happen. This means that if you happen to take the emergency contraceptive pill after you ovulate, it can't exactly do its job. This doesn't mean you will definitely become pregnant; an egg only survives around twenty-four hours after ovulation so this window may have already passed. It also isn't to say that you shouldn't take the emergency contraceptive pill. The reality is that most people can't be sure when they've ovulated and the emergency contraceptive pill is incredibly safe to take regardless. It's completely false to say that the emergency contraceptive pill is an abortifacient (abortion pill), as the hormones don't affect an egg that's already been released and fertilised. Unfortunately, this is a misconception that's often spread by abortion groups.

Some medications can interfere with the effectiveness of

the emergency contraceptive pill (though this doesn't mean you can't use it). If you're taking any other medications, including over-the-counter remedies and any herbal ones, be sure to let your healthcare professional know. This is particularly important if you have severe asthma, use epilepsy medication, have HIV or tuberculosis, are taking certain antibiotics, use St John's wort or take medication for stomach acid. ellaOne may not work if you're already taking one of these medicines but you can use the copper IUD or the levonorgestrel pill (your healthcare professional may advise doubling the dose).

Research published in 2023 found that taking the emergency contraceptive pill with the painkiller piroxicam is more effective than taking the emergency contraceptive pill alone.[4] This is because piroxicam reduces the release of chemicals called prostaglandins which help support ovulation and fertilisation of the egg. At the time of writing, the findings of this study haven't led to piroxicam being prescribed alongside the emergency contraceptive pill, as more investigation is needed. It is a potentially exciting development, though, and we'd love to see more research into emergency contraception and how it can serve users better!

---

**Q:** Can you overdose on the morning after pill? I've been advised to take two because of my BMI.

**A:** You may be advised to take two doses of the levonorgestrel emergency contraceptive pill if you have a BMI over 26 or weigh over 70 kg or if you take other medication which could interact with it (though a double dose of ellaOne isn't recommended). Always stick to the dose advised by your doctor or pharmacist. Taking more pills than you need doesn't mean you're more likely to prevent pregnancy. In fact, it could actually have an adverse effect as you may end up vomiting, which can make the emergency contraceptive pill less effective.

---

*How will you know if the emergency contraceptive pill has worked?*

It's recommended that you take a pregnancy test three weeks after taking the emergency contraceptive pill. Don't rely on bleeding as a sign you're not pregnant, as the emergency contraceptive pill itself can affect your period, or cause spotting or bleeding. The emergency contraceptive pill itself can affect the timings of your period, making it late, so try not to worry if it doesn't arrive on time. Keep reading to find out why this is.

*Accessing emergency contraceptive pills*

Your GP, pharmacy or sexual health clinic can supply emergency contraception. It's important to contact them ASAP to get an appointment as you only have a small window in which to use it to prevent pregnancy. In the UK, you can get it for free from most GP surgeries or NHS sexual health clinics and from some pharmacies. There's also the option of buying it from a pharmacy (which is sometimes speedier). At the time of writing, we're also hearing of efforts to try to get both types of emergency contraceptive pill available in shops (like supermarkets and garages) so that you don't need to speak to a pharmacist before purchasing. We think this would be a great step to provide an extremely convenient way to access these pills at all times, and hope to see this change happen.

We surveyed 2,658 women to ask who pays when they

buy the emergency contraceptive pill; 33 per cent said they did, 12 per cent said their sexual partner did and 55 per cent said they split the cost equally.[5] What would you do?

**Lowdown life hack**

Lots of people don't know this, but you can actually buy the emergency contraceptive pill even if you don't need it, to keep as a spare for emergencies. It saves a few hours of frantic googling for your nearest out-of-hours pharmacy, clinic or GP surgery – because it always seems to be a bank holiday weekend when these things happen. Speak to your GP, sexual health clinic or pharmacist to see if this is an option they offer.

*Side effects*

The emergency contraceptive pill is generally very safe and there are no serious or long-term side effects associated with it. In fact, most people don't feel any side effects when taking it, though some may experience nausea, vomiting, headache or stomach aches. It's important to remember that if you vomit within three hours of taking an emergency contraceptive pill,[6] you'll need to make another visit to the pharmacy or clinic to get a second dose or to consider the emergency copper IUD.

Some people find that the emergency contraceptive pill makes their skin worse after taking it, but this won't happen to everyone. The most common side effect of using the emergency contraceptive pill includes a temporary impact on your menstrual cycle. It can cause your period to be longer, shorter, heavier, lighter, earlier or delayed ... you get the gist. This is because the emergency contraceptive pill delays ovulation and, as a result, alters the timings of your natural cycle. All of these changes should only last for one cycle before your period returns to your 'normal'. If you take the emergency contraceptive pill this could affect fertility tracking. Your fertile days in your next cycle may be different to what you might usually expect. You may also experience some spotting or irregular bleeding if you've taken the emergency contraceptive pill while getting back on track with your usual hormonal contraception.

**Morning after pill**
28 years old

★★★★☆

**Levonorgestrel pill**

I've been using the morning after pill which has most definitely been very effective for me. I don't really experience any excessive side effects but what I do notice every time I take this medication my period comes a week later than normal and it can be much heavier at times with more clots, and the periods are very painful.

Shared on **thelowdown.com**

---

**Q:** If I take the morning after pill too many times, will I become infertile?

**A:** This is one of the most common myths we hear of when it comes to the emergency contraceptive pill, likely because so many people don't know that all it does is delay ovulation.

It's another glaring gap in women's health knowledge that isn't deemed essential to teach us in schools, and there's an incredible amount of scaremongering around it. But no, there is no limit to the number of times you can take the emergency contraceptive pill, or how often you can take it. You can even take it multiple times in one menstrual cycle if you need to but speak to a healthcare professional in this case. You should stick to the same type of emergency contraceptive pill in the same cycle as levonorgestrel and ulipristal acetate work differently and may interfere with each other, which could reduce their effectiveness. Both types of emergency contraceptive pill have no long-term effects on your body, and won't cause any fertility problems. The reason that it's not recommended you take it too often is simply because it's not as reliable as an ongoing contraceptive method.

---

**Q:** Can I take the morning after pill if I'm breastfeeding?

**A:** Yes! If you are breastfeeding and want to use emergency contraception, you can now choose any option, remembering that the copper coil is the most effective.

The hormone from the levonorgestrel pill can be found in breast milk in tiny amounts, but there's no evidence that there are any harmful side effects for babies.

Despite the patient information leaflet in levonorgestrel pills advising that you may want to wait eight hours after taking the pill to breastfeed again, the Breastfeeding Network say that there's no evidence to support this.[7] This just goes to show that more research is sorely needed when it comes to drugs, pregnancy and breastfeeding.

Guidance from 2025[8] states that ellaOne is also safe to take while breastfeeding. Previously, you were advised to not breastfeed for seven days after taking ellaOne,[9] but new research has shown that such a negligible amount of the drug is found in breastmilk, it is safe to take. If you have any further worries or questions about breastfeeding, see our Resources section for breastfeeding support.

---

*Starting contraception after taking the emergency contraceptive pill*

If you're currently using hormonal contraception but needed the emergency contraceptive pill due to an accident or other issue (like a missed pill, delayed injection or vomiting), you can continue with your current method. The levonorgestrel pill doesn't affect your contraceptive so just keep on using it as normal. However, if you've chosen to use ellaOne, you should delay restarting or stop using hormonal contraception for five days afterwards. This is because the progestin in your contraceptive can actually stop ellaOne from working effectively.

You should use condoms or abstain from sex for the five days after taking ellaOne, and then you can restart your hormonal contraception. For the traditional or desogestrel-based progestogen-only pills, you need to use condoms or avoid sex for two days after starting them. For every other method, it's seven days.[10]

You're advised to take a pregnancy test three weeks after unprotected sex to check whether the emergency contraceptive pill has worked. You don't need to delay starting hormonal contraception during these three weeks as the available evidence shows that there is no harmful effect of hormones from contraception on an early pregnancy.

## Emergency contraceptive options compared

| | **Levonorgestrel emergency contraceptive pill** |
|---|---|
| **Type** | Hormonal pill containing levonorgestrel |
| **Rough cost, if you're buying from a pharmacy (it is free via prescription from your GP)** | £3–£5 upwards |
| **Works up to ...** | 3 days (72 hours) after unprotected sex |
| **May not be suitable if you ...** | - Have a BMI over 26 or weigh more than 70kg, consider taking two pills at the same time |

## Unintended pregnancy

If you've missed the window to use emergency contraception, or you didn't realise your contraception had failed and find that you are now pregnant – don't panic. There is no one right course of action to take if you discover you're unexpectedly pregnant, and it's normal to feel a range of emotions. Whatever you decide, there's support out there to help you.

### You're pregnant. What next?

• **'Wow, I wasn't expecting this but, actually, I'm feeling pretty happy about it!'** If you accidentally get pregnant and feel pleased, then congratulations! First, you should start taking vitamin D and folic acid, cut out alcohol and stop

| ellaOne emergency contraceptive pill | Copper coil (IUD) |
|---|---|
| Hormonal pill containing ulipristal acetate | Non-hormonal coil, fitted inside the uterus |
| £16–£20 upwards | You can't buy this in a pharmacy – and will need to find a sexual health clinic or GP to fit this for you. In the UK this will be free |
| 5 days (120 hours) after unprotected sex | 5 days (120 hours) after unprotected sex or up to 5 days after you have ovulated – whichever is later |
| - Have used hormonal contraception in the last 7 days<br>- Have severe asthma | - Don't want to have a coil fitted |

smoking. Contact your GP, who will loop you in with your local midwife team and check you're taking the right folic acid dose. See our Resources for more on how to keep healthy during pregnancy, including info on how to boost your well-being and what to avoid.

- **'I'm totally overwhelmed and don't know what to do'** It's normal to resemble the head-exploding emoji in this situation. Go for a walk to clear your head, and avoid rushing into a decision. Consider speaking to someone you trust and/or a counselling service that is impartial and non-judgemental (see our UK-based recommendations in the Resources). Sometimes just talking through the options can help bring clarity to the situation. It may be a good idea to follow the health and supplement advice in the previous section too, until you are sure what you'd like to do.
- **'I don't want to have a baby right now'** If you don't want

or aren't able to have a child (or another one) at this stage in your life, your options are abortion (termination of pregnancy) or adoption after delivery. Adoption is sometimes chosen by those who have gone beyond the legal date for an abortion, or those who do not want to have a termination. With adoption, after the birth, you hand over the legal rights and responsibilities for the child, which are then passed on to the adoptive family. The whole process is arranged by adoption agencies or a local authority.

## Abortion

Abortion is a medical (using tablets) or surgical procedure to end a pregnancy, also known as a termination. Abortion is really common – one in three women in the UK will have one before they're forty-five,[11] for a whole host of reasons. Women, trans men and non-binary people from all backgrounds, religions, ethnicities, marital status and age groups undergo abortions. While teenage abortion rates have been on the decline for the last decade, the number of over-thirty-fives having terminations is increasing.[12] Procedures are carried out in NHS hospitals or licensed clinics, and medication can be taken in your own home.

Abortions are generally very safe and serious complications are uncommon. Though much of the info in this upcoming section is with unintended pregnancy in mind, abortions are also carried out for medical reasons, known as TFMR (terminating a pregnancy for medical reasons). There may be a number of causes, such as if tests indicate the foetus isn't developing as it should or if pregnancy complications put the mother's or baby's health at risk. If you're having a termination for this reason, you will be advised on your options by your medical team. It can be a very difficult decision for parents to make and there are organisations that can offer support (see Antenatal Results and Choices in Resources). Whatever your reasons for seeking a termination, you should feel supported every step of the way.

Access to abortion services is completely confidential. Healthcare professionals will only share information about you if they have reason to be concerned that you, or anyone else, is at risk of harm. Even if you're under sixteen. As long as you understand all of the advice about abortion and its implications, and it is in your best interests to have treatment without your parents knowing, then your healthcare professional will not tell them. You will be asked if you would like to tell your parents, but if you don't, that's your choice.

---

**Q:** Will having an abortion impact my chances of having a healthy pregnancy down the road?

**A:** No, it will rarely have any bearing on your fertility or subsequent pregnancies. The only exception to this is a rare complication after a surgical abortion called Asherman's syndrome, which occurs in around 1.6 per cent of surgical abortions.[13] This can cause scar tissue to form in the uterus which can affect fertility. However, this isn't seen in medical abortions (where medication is used to end the pregnancy), which make up 86 per cent of abortions.[14]

---

## Accessing abortion services

When Roe vs. Wade was overturned in the US in 2022, it was a shocking reminder of how abortion rights legislation can be snatched away overnight. The right to abortion care is under threat in many parts of the world, and the legalities surrounding it vary from country to country. Abortion is an important part of healthcare, but it's become a highly politicised debate, with most anti-abortionist groups placing more rights on an unborn foetus over the person whose body it resides in. At the time of writing, abortion is only legal in the UK if it has been allowed by the signatures of two doctors; otherwise, it is still a crime as dictated by the Abortion Act of 1967, although this continues to teeter on the edge of debate in Parliament. Abortion was fully decriminalised in Northern Ireland in 2019 and many other countries are following suit to modernise abortion care.

In 2022, we surveyed over 500 women about their abortion experience; 40 per cent rated the information and advice they received about their different options, and how to choose between them, as 'average'. Only 26 per cent rated it 'very good', while 17 per cent rated it 'poor'.[15] We want to demystify what happens during the abortion process, not only so that you feel more prepared if you ever need to access one, but also so you can empathise and support anyone close to you who might have one.

Firstly, if you do need to arrange an abortion you can phone your GP or visit a sexual health clinic, who will refer you to your local NHS abortion service. Or you can self-refer to some NHS services, a private clinic or charity (see the Resources section). Private clinics are government-regulated, safe and confidential and 99 per cent of people will get the treatment paid for by the NHS.[16]

In the UK, the vast majority of abortions are performed within the first twelve weeks of pregnancy. There are two main types of abortion: medical (i.e. taking medication that ends the pregnancy) or surgical (having the pregnancy removed from the body). The method you have will depend on the number of weeks pregnant you are, your suitability, as well as your preference. If you are less than ten weeks pregnant, you may be able to access the 'pills by post' scheme. This involves having a phone or video consultation with a specialist and based on their assessment, you may be able to have a medical abortion at home.

If it's deemed that you need to be seen in-person, you should be given an appointment within one week of referral. A healthcare professional (usually a specialist nurse) will talk through your options and check you're happy with your decision. You'll be offered further counselling if you are still not sure, but this is not compulsory. A medical assessment may be carried out which can involve:

- An ultrasound scan to see how many weeks pregnant you are. This may need to be with a small probe inserted into your vagina if the pregnancy is very early. Ultrasounds are not needed for everyone and you do not have to watch the scan if you do not want to.
- A blood test to check your blood type.
- Swabs to check for sexually transmitted infections (STIs). This is to ensure if you do have an STI you receive prompt treatment in order to reduce the risk of complications. This is because some STIs can travel from the vagina to the uterus during an abortion procedure, and increase the risk of post-abortion infections.

Following this, you and a healthcare professional will discuss the best option for your abortion procedure, which should be scheduled to take place within one week of your referral appointment. You can change your mind at any time, including right up until before the procedure starts.

Of the people we surveyed about their abortion experience, 51 per cent said that knowing what to expect beforehand would have improved their overall experience, which is why we've included descriptions of what happens during each kind of abortion in this next section. As the anonymous responses to our survey indicate (you'll find those responses dotted throughout this chapter), many women find this experience incredibly difficult . . .

> *'I felt ashamed, alone and confused about the procedure. I went in with very little information and out with none. I kept it a secret from everybody despite being incredibly unwell for two weeks.'*

### Medical abortion

This is the most common method of abortion, with 86 per cent of people choosing this in 2022.[17] As we've explained, if you're less than ten weeks pregnant, you may be able to have a medical abortion at home. Research studies have shown that it is safe and effective to have an abortion at home, they work and they are acceptable for women.[18]

From weeks ten to twenty-four, a termination will always be overseen in a hospital or clinic. It's carried out using two tablets taken twenty-four to forty-eight hours apart. The first, mifepristone, ends the pregnancy; the second, misoprostol, opens the cervix (neck of the uterus) and causes the uterus to contract so the pregnancy is passed out of the vagina.

You should expect to start bleeding within two to four hours of taking the second tablet. If not, you may need more medication – this will be explained clearly before you start the treatment. Usually, you will pass large blood clots, which is the pregnancy leaving your body. These shouldn't be larger than the size of a lemon. In most cases, you cannot see a recognisable foetus within this pregnancy tissue.

> *'My body was so sore and nobody told me this would happen. I was feeling pretty low about the situation as my friends were not as supportive but I had a very supportive partner and therapist at the time. It really helped being able to take the abortion at home.'*

If you're at home, you can either flush this down the toilet or wrap it in tissue and put it in a normal household bin inside a plastic bag. In the hospital, the pregnancy tissue will be collected and it is your choice whether you take this home or leave it at the hospital. You'll be advised to use sanitary towels rather than tampons or a menstrual cup to track your bleeding. Most abortions are complete within one to two days and your bleeding should become lighter after the pregnancy has passed. However, sometimes the bleeding can go on for up to two weeks.

> *'I felt wiped out, the fairy tale of women being at work while their body is going through a medical abortion is wild.'*

## Surgical abortion

In 2022, 14 per cent of women had a surgical abortion – which is the name for an abortion that involves a minor operation, carried out by an experienced gynaecology doctor.[19] There are two types: vacuum aspiration, and dilation and evacuation.

- **Vacuum aspiration** This is an option if you are fourteen weeks pregnant or less. It works by removing the pregnancy using gentle suction. You may be offered the procedure using local anaesthetic, which could shorten your recovery time and how long you have to stay in the clinic. Sedation or general anaesthetic might also be offered.

• **Dilation and evacuation** This is the option if you are fourteen to twenty-four weeks pregnant. Forceps are used to remove the pregnancy through the neck of the uterus, Depending on the number of weeks you are pregnant, general anaesthetic or sedation will be given.

## What happens after an abortion?

- Pregnancy sickness and nausea should stop within one to two days, but sore boobs may continue for up to three weeks.
- If you are over ten weeks pregnant and your blood tests show that your blood type is Rhesus D negative, it's recommended you have an injection to prevent complications in subsequent pregnancies.[20]
- You can have sex when you feel ready to, but be mindful of infection and also consider your contraceptive options if required. You can ovulate as early as eight days after an abortion.[21]
- You can go swimming as soon as the pregnancy has passed – the burning question on everyone's mind, we're sure.
- You should avoid alcohol for twenty-four hours after the abortion but drink plenty of water.
- Your vagina will clean itself naturally using its own discharge, so don't use douches or intimate washes.
- If you're breastfeeding, you can continue to feed as normal. The medications used in a medical abortion do not transfer into milk, and even if you have a general anaesthetic, breastfeeding experts agree it's fine to feed after.[22]

- After three weeks, you should take a pregnancy test. If you do one too early, it might still be positive. If it's positive after three weeks – get in touch with your clinic.

## Side effects

We asked women what kinds of symptoms or issues they experienced after having an abortion. Here's what they said:

**Which of these things did you experience during or after your abortion?**

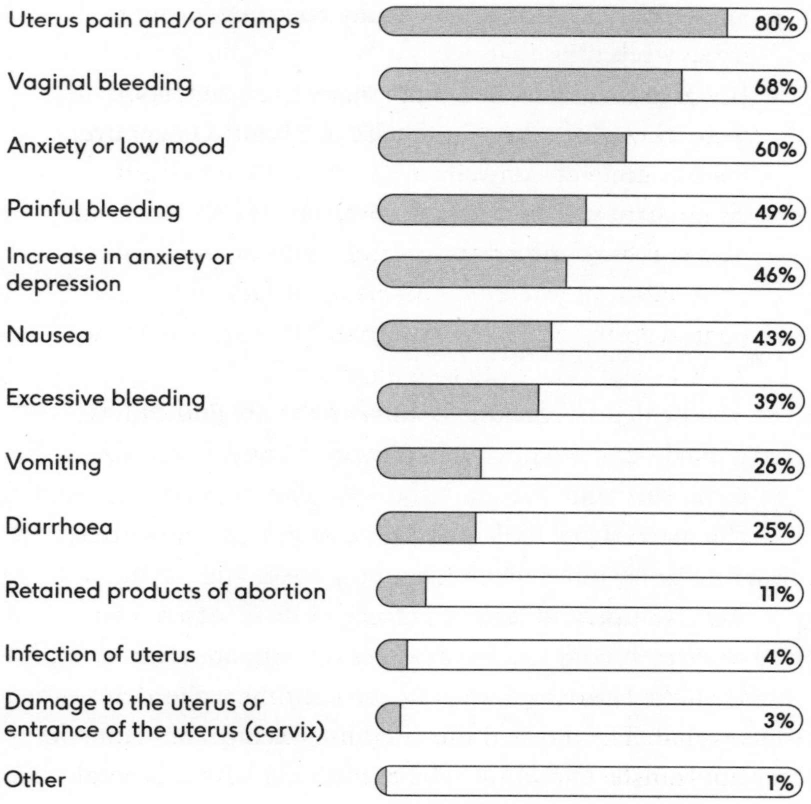


556 people answered this question (with multiple choice)

### Risks

There are some rare risks associated with abortion, and you should be aware of the signs so you know when to get help:

- Infection can cause a fever, smelly vaginal discharge or ongoing pain and bleeding – ring your clinic for help if you experience any of these.
- Failed abortion is when the procedure hasn't worked and you don't pass the pregnancy, which can be really upsetting. If this happens, call your clinic.
- Heavy bleeding that needs a blood transfusion. If you are bleeding through a pad every thirty minutes, call your clinic for advice and help, or 999 if you are dizzy, pale or feel very unwell.
- Surgical abortion also has a very small risk of damage to the cervix and uterus.

### How might you feel afterwards?

Any medical procedure can cause anxiety and an abortion particularly can take its toll physically and psychologically. For some, the time after an abortion can be a bit of an emotional rollercoaster. A lot of the responses to our survey on abortion mention feeling numb, guilty and struggling to process emotions as feelings changed quite often in the first weeks after having it. It isn't helped that abortion is still a taboo subject in wider society (something we're determined to help change). Many of the responses to our abortion survey mention a mix of feeling relieved but emotionally impacted. So many of the responses to our survey talk about secrecy, shame and feeling judged.

*'I was relieved to have my body back and felt lucky to have had the option. But I was shocked by the emotional impact – I always knew I didn't want kids so thought it would be an easy decision. I wasn't prepared for the guilt, shame and grief of losing something I didn't even want.'*

While it can be a really emotionally draining process, not everyone who goes through an abortion will find it to be traumatic. For example, here are a few of the responses to our survey question: 'What do you wish you'd known before having an abortion?':

*'That all the myths about pain, regret and possible trauma were not true (for all women). I was made to believe an abortion was going to be painful, traumatising and stressful. But it was OK. It was fine. The people working at the clinic were amazing, I felt fine afterwards and it was done quickly.'*

*'I wish I had general knowledge of good or positive abortion stories before I got to a point where I needed one. The general discourse is scaremongering and it meant that I was initially panicked by my pregnancy. Had I known that abortion could be a positive, unstigmatised experience, I would have felt less daunted by the option.'*

Of the people we surveyed about their abortion experience, the majority said that while they were told about the physical symptoms to expect after their termination, there was a lack of support around the emotional side effects: 29 per cent rated their aftercare and support as 'poor' and another 29 per cent rated it 'average', while 24 per cent rated it 'terrible'.[23]

Hopefully, you will have support from a partner, family or friends. But if not, there are organisations (see Resources) that can provide a listening ear if you'd like to talk it out. It may be really helpful to speak to people who have been through a similar experience. Being in a safe space to explore your feelings and process your experience can be really cathartic.

### Contraception while waiting for an abortion

If you're already using a method of contraception and accidentally fall pregnant – what on earth do you do about it while waiting for an abortion? The implant and injection can just be continued as usual throughout and after the abortion, as long as they are within their expiry date. If you're using a pill, patch or ring, these should be stopped then started again immediately after the procedure. Coils should be removed if you are under twelve weeks pregnant, but can be immediately replaced after the abortion is completed.[24]

### Fertility and contraception after an abortion

You are potentially fertile almost immediately after an abortion. One study showed 90 per cent of women released an egg within one month of the procedure.[25] So, you may want to start thinking about contraception going forward. This will be discussed at your appointment, and even if you are having an abortion at home, contraception can be delivered to your door. If you do want to get pregnant again, some providers advise to wait until after your next period to start trying to conceive again.

All forms of contraception can be started safely after an abortion. The progestogen-only pill, implant and injection can even be started when you have the first abortion pill (although having the injection can increase your risk of having a failed abortion). The combined pill, patch or ring can be started immediately after an abortion. The copper or hormonal coil can be inserted after a pregnancy has passed (unless there is an infection). You don't need to use any extra protection if contraception is started within five days of the abortion. If you have been using fertility awareness methods, be aware that they may be less reliable after an abortion while your cycle gets into a rhythm again, and if using a diaphragm, your diaphragm size may have changed so it's worth getting this checked.

## Legislation changes to decriminalise abortion

Abortion is an area of healthcare that can be deeply emotive and very divisive. Different countries vary on their abortion policies, and in some parts of the world access to abortion is illegal or extremely limited. UK laws are linked to pregnancy timing and certain medical circumstances.

Abortion law dates back to the 1800s and states that abortion in the UK is illegal. With the 1967 Abortion Act, abortion became legal but only if it is performed by a doctor and authorised by two doctors who agree the pregnancy has not exceeded twenty-four weeks, or if over twenty-four weeks is necessary on medical grounds (to prevent serious permanent injury to the physical or mental health of the pregnant woman or risk to her life, or if the child were born it would suffer from such physical or mental abnormalities as to be seriously disabled). It also has to be carried out in an NHS setting or somewhere that has been approved by the Secretary of State (thanks to COVID, your own home is now approved).

Any abortions that take place beyond these parameters are considered a criminal offence. This means women (and sometimes men) are prosecuted under the 'Offences Against the Person Act' of 1861, a time before women were even allowed to vote or set foot in Parliament where laws were being made.[26] This same archaic law dictates that a woman should be 'kept in penal servitude for life' if she is found guilty.

We believe that abortion should be completely decriminalised, both across the whole of the UK and across the world. Access to safe and legal abortion healthcare is a fundamental right, for whatever reason you may need one. Many of the women who have faced prosecution under this law are already living vulnerable lives. There have been incidents of women being arrested at their hospital bed for suspected illegal abortion and even cases of women who have had stillbirths (due to natural causes) being under criminal investigation. The reality is that the criminality of later-term abortion can leave women with no choice but to obtain abortions in an unsafe way that may cause harm.

It seems right that people should be shown compassion in these circumstances, rather than punishment. We need to see more investment into good health provision and less energy spent stigmatising or politicising abortion. Adequate funding for this key area of women's health needs to be prioritised so that those accessing abortion services can be seen and treated without delay.

# 9

# Planning for pregnancy

For years, you've likely been diligent about *not* getting pregnant – it's no surprise, as most of us had school sex education that only focused on STIs and warnings around teen pregnancy. For so long the people around us were telling us not to get pregnant, then suddenly it's like, 'So, when are you going to have a baby?' For others, it's as though an internal switch gets flicked, from 'Must not get pregnant' to 'I need to get pregnant now'. Equally, remember, that if someone tells you they're pregnant you might only be getting the tip of the iceberg – below the surface there may have been months or years of trying.

This chapter is all about what happens after you stop using contraception, what the science says about fertility and how to prepare your body as best you can for pregnancy. We'll be casting an eye on what can impact fertility and interventions that are sometimes taken when it's not the simplest journey. If you're curious about your fertility or coming off your method to try for a baby, this chapter has got you covered.

While we discuss natural family planning and assisted conception in this chapter, there is more than one route to starting a family – from co-parenting, fostering and adoption to surrogacy and more. If you're interested in finding out more about creating your family through any of these pathways, there are lots of helpful organisations out there (see Resources).

## Not everyone's fertility journey is the same

Looking into your fertility, deciding to have a child and then trying to conceive is a highly personal journey – and it doesn't necessarily go in that order. We've learnt first-hand that lots of people simply don't talk about it. In 2023, we ran a survey that asked over 500 women what their fertility journey was like, and the response was, overwhelmingly, 'lonely'. More than one in three women hadn't told anyone except for their partner that they are or were trying to conceive, even though 48 per cent said that they would want to hear other women's stories.[1]

We found that there was a huge gap in knowledge around how long it can take to conceive, which led to almost half of respondents saying that trying to conceive has taken 'longer' or 'much longer' than expected. This is despite the fact that the majority of respondents (58 per cent) had only been trying for one to three months so far, or had gotten pregnant within three months. We also found that not knowing why trying to conceive wasn't working (45 per cent), alongside mixed feelings about friends and family getting pregnant around them (50 per cent) and not knowing when they had ovulated (41 per cent) were key sources of uncertainty around the whole process.[2]

It's no wonder women feel lonely, frustrated and unable to talk about their fertility journey when they don't feel like they have all the facts. If your loved ones are getting pregnant and you're still trying, it can feel like there's something wrong with you, or that you're 'failing' somehow. This is categorically not the case. How long it takes you to conceive, or whether you're able to conceive at all, is not on you. While there are many factors that can help boost or reduce fertility, there are some things which are totally out of your control. To help people going through this experience, we launched an area on The Lowdown website where you can share your experiences with trying to conceive.

**Fertility experience**

Trying for 6 months    33 years old

When my husband and I decided to go for it and try for a baby, we really didn't know how long it would take, but both felt that it was definitely something we wanted. Trying to conceive was exciting, but also nerve racking (what if it didn't work, what would that mean?), and also a bit all-consuming and lonely at times. I told a few close friends that we were thinking about having kids, but didn't really discuss it in depth with anyone, especially as we were the first in our friendship group to say that 'we felt ready' for children. On reflection, I wish I'd been more open with some of my friends that we were trying. I actually listened to a couple of podcasts about trying to conceive and IVF, which I found really comforting but also fun and informative. I ended up falling pregnant in a couple of months and was over the moon when I got the positive test (albeit slightly surprised it has happened so quickly!), but felt very fortunate. I used Natural Cycles to help me understand when I was ovulating, and therefore the best time for my husband and I to have sex. The app is super-easy to use – I had previously used it for birth control and switched to the 'plan pregnancy' mode. I also used LH ovulation tests, which I found useful to use in tandem with the app.

Shared on **thelowdown.com**

## Fertility 101

What do we actually mean when we talk about 'fertility'? Well, fertility is simply the ability to conceive a child. We say 'simply', but as you're three-quarters of the way through reading this book, you'll know human biology is often not that 'simple'. Let's recap the basics ... You'll remember from Chapter 1 that to conceive, an egg released from the ovaries needs to be fertilised by sperm. If you've been using any form of contraception in the past, it'll have been working to prevent this from happening. If you have ovaries, you are born with all your eggs, you don't make any more. Our egg supply gradually depletes as we age, with many people experiencing a big decrease in the quality and quantity of their eggs from their mid to late thirties and early forties. By the time menopause occurs (more on that in Chapter 11) it's no longer possible to get pregnant naturally.

If you decide to try for a baby, unfortunately, there's no way to predict how long it'll take to get pregnant. For some couples (a lucky 30 per cent),[3] it happens the first month they try, while others conceive after months or years of trying. It can also vary a lot for couples who have subsequent children; for example, even if it took years of trying for one baby, it can happen much more quickly for another. Some people might try to 'schedule' a baby to arrive at the 'perfect' time of year, but honestly, that's quite hard to do. It may well happen, or life may have other plans in store. How long it takes you to conceive isn't easy to predict, and it's not a failing on your part if you're unable to conceive as quickly as you'd like, or at all. If you take anything away from this chapter, we hope it's that.

**Fertility experience**

Trying for 1–3 years    32 years old

It's been very hard, much harder than I ever imagined, mostly because after a year it still hasn't happened. I hoped that after coming off the pill (Cerelle), which I had taken for thirteen years, I'd fall pregnant in the first three months, you're taught at school that unprotected sex leads to pregnancy. In those first three months of trying my expectations were high and they were very difficult months when it didn't happen. Three to six months of trying were hard too. The negative pregnancy tests, the PMS symptoms, which are similar to early pregnancy symptoms, getting your hopes up and a period arriving and tearing down all the hope from that month. We went to see the doctor early, at six months [of trying to conceive], as my periods are very light and only last three days (prior to the pill I was on medication for heavy periods and my heavy periods were the reason I was put on the pill). The first doctor I saw didn't treat me very well – he dismissed me, told us it hadn't been a year yet. But I persevered, knowing something wasn't right. Eventually a different doctor listened to me and an internal scan and blood tests confirmed I don't ovulate, have no endometrial lining and low progesterone. Then my husband's semen analysis came back with problems too and we were referred to the local fertility clinic, with a four-month waiting list to be seen. We've been told that we won't conceive unless we have IVF. I feel like my body is failing me, that others seem to get pregnant so easily, and mostly I feel that it's unfair. Being told we needed IVF was the biggest blow as it was like all the endless monthly chances I thought we had are now vastly reduced to one round of IVF that we are entitled to on the NHS, unless we want to and can afford to pay for more treatment privately. And there's a long wait first to even get to that one chance.

Shared on **thelowdown.com**

## Fertility after contraception

You'll probably be wondering about your fertility when you stop your contraceptive method in the hope of conceiving. This is something we get asked about *a lot* at The Lowdown, and we can confirm that there are multiple studies and decades of research to show that hormonal contraception does not impact your long-term fertility. The length of time you used it, whether you took a monthly break on the combined pill and whether or not you had withdrawal bleeds while using it have no impact. When you stop using your method, your fertility will return to whatever is normal for you. So, your ability to get pregnant will be the same whether or not you have used hormonal contraception, keeping in mind that fertility declines as we get older.

Let's say you've stopped using your method in the hope of getting pregnant, now what? In theory, it's possible to get pregnant pretty much as soon as you stop taking hormonal contraception. As per Chapter 7, with most hormonal methods, most users find their period returns to what's normal for them within one to three months of stopping. While having periods does not necessarily indicate fertility (it's possible not to ovulate every cycle, see page 22), studies show the majority of women do ovulate within a month of stopping most hormonal methods.[4]

The only exception to this is the injection (e.g. the Depo Provera or Sayana Press), which has the longest potential delay before your baseline fertility returns.[5] For some it can take twelve to eighteen months from your last injection for your cycle to return to normal (though this is only for a minority). The injection works by stopping ovulation, and a common side effect is changes to your bleeding pattern, including stopping bleeding completely. It can take a while for your period and ovulation to return once you stop having injections.

Though you may experience irregular cycles after stopping the injection, you may still ovulate (it's just sometimes more difficult to keep track of when ovulation occurs). It's really important to remember that this delay, however frustrating, is transient. Research shows that over 80 per cent of women trying to conceive may expect to become pregnant within fifteen months of their last Depo-Provera injection,[6] and after two years there is no significant difference in pregnancy rates compared with users of non-hormonal contraception.[7] This might seem a long time, though, if you're desperate to have a baby. With this in mind, if you would like to fall pregnant in the reasonably near future, you might want to consider stopping the injection, and switching to another method in the short term if you don't want to conceive straight away.

## Trying to get pregnant

While we can't control every aspect of our fertility, what we do know is that there are things we can do to give us the best shot at conceiving. Let's look at some of these measures – both for men and women. There are also issues that can make it harder to get pregnant, such as underlying medical conditions, which we'll dive into on page 270.

### How long will it take to get pregnant?

As we've already seen, we'd love to be able to give an answer to this much-asked question, but the truth is it varies between individuals. It's normal for around 80 per cent of couples with no fertility problems to take up to twelve months to conceive; 46 per cent of couples with mild fertility problems and 11 per cent of couples with severe fertility problems will get pregnant naturally within twelve months.[8]

## What do you need to know if you want to get pregnant now or in the future?

Whether you are baby-ready or simply fertility-curious (i.e. you know you want kids eventually, or are open to the idea), you might be wondering what you can do now to improve your fertility. Taking practical measures for your day-to-day well-being can in turn help your fertility in the long and short run. It's never too early to adopt lifestyle changes even if you are still using contraception, and all of these measures will improve your overall health, even if you're not planning on impending parenthood. As well as all the usual recommendations from healthcare professionals, we'll look at some lesser-known things that can impact or improve fertility, and how all of these recommendations are linked to fertility in the first place.

*First, the basics*

- **Come off contraception** (duh, but hear us out). Coming off contraception can be as simple as no longer taking it, or making an appointment with a healthcare professional to have it removed. But as we discussed in Chapter 7, it's important to know how stopping hormonal contraception can temporarily affect things like your menstrual cycle, and whether it might unmask an underlying condition. In Chapter 4, we saw how contraception can be really effective at managing the symptoms of conditions like polycystic ovary syndrome (PCOS) and endometriosis, which can also make it harder to become pregnant. If you're concerned about heavy, painful or irregular periods, or any other unusual symptoms when you come off your contraception, speak to a healthcare professional. We'll look at PCOS and endometriosis again in more detail later in this chapter, and how they can impact fertility.

• **Have sex, a lot** It's recommended you have unprotected penetrative penis-in-vagina sex every two to three days while trying to conceive. Sperm can survive inside the female reproductive tract for up to five days (thanks, sperm crypts), and regular sex will boost the chances of sperm still hanging around during ovulation and your fertile window. FYI, it's totally normal for sex to start feeling more like a chore than something to look forward to if you're actively trying to conceive. While some people find that scheduling sex helps, it can also take some of the spontaneity out of it for sure. Try to break the boredom by scheduling date nights, engaging in non-sexual physical contact like the humble cuddle or having a different type of sex on the days when you're less likely to be fertile.

**The lifecycle of sperm**

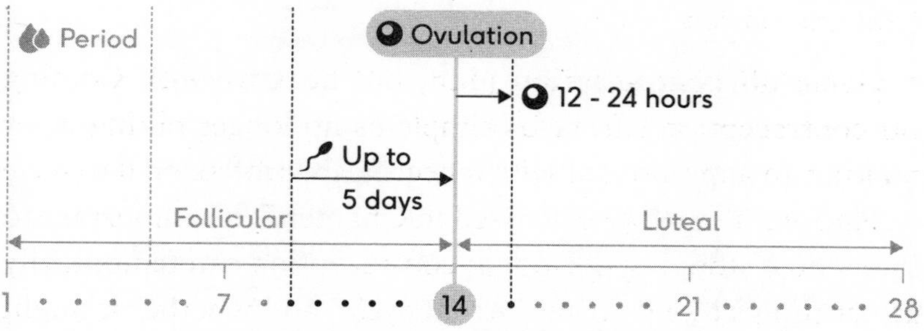


Days of the menstrual cycle

• **Know your cycle** From subtle changes in your temperature to the changing consistency of your cervical fluid and even ovulation discomfort or pain for some, knowing when you're most fertile is key to boosting your chances of conceiving. Additionally, if you notice your periods are irregular, it can be harder to know when you're ovulating and when your best chance of conceiving that month is. You can speak to a

**Fertility experience**

Trying for 1 year    34 years old

It took seven months to conceive with my first. It was tough as everyone around me was seeming to get pregnant immediately, including friends and family members. Sex became boring and stressful and my husband wasn't enjoying it. This was also mid-lockdown 2020 and our wedding had been postponed. It was really strange being happy for people announcing their pregnancies while also feeling upset, angry and jealous and not being able to control those feelings – feelings that I now know are common in people [tying to conceive] but just not talked about!

After the first six months I decided to give up, as it didn't feel like it was working. We got married and I drank loads of alcohol. Then the next month I felt really flu-like and tired and just knew it was different. I was late by one to two days so decided to do a test and it was positive! We'd only had sex twice that month! I know that stress isn't meant to play a part in getting pregnant but I definitely feel like it was for me. It wasn't until I stopped caring or being obsessed that it happened. Second time round was completely different – I noticed my vaginal discharge was sticky and fertile, drank too much wine and was pregnant before we'd even started trying properly! Probably because I was relaxed, my body knew what it was doing this time and I knew how to recognise my fertile signs.

Shared on **thelowdown.com**

healthcare professional about this, or even try wearable ovulation tracking devices that track subtle temperature changes.

*Next, the health stuff*

- **Folic acid** In the UK, the advice for anyone trying to get pregnant is to take 400 micrograms of folic acid every day from at least three months *before* you start trying to get pregnant and up until twelve weeks of pregnancy. This is because folic acid can help prevent conditions such as spina bifida, which can occur during the baby's development in the early weeks of pregnancy. If you have a higher chance of your pregnancy being affected by these types of birth defects (for instance, if your BMI is over 30, you have diabetes, sickle cell disease or take anti-epilepsy medications), you will need to take a higher dose of 5 milligrams of folic acid, which is prescribed via your GP.
- **Vitamins** In the UK, pregnant and breastfeeding mothers are advised to take 10 micrograms of vitamin D every day to support the development of bones, teeth and muscles. Don't take a vitamin A supplement (or multivitamins that contain it) or other supplements such as cod liver oil, as it can be potentially harmful to a developing baby.
- **Prescribed medication, over-the-counter treatments and herbal remedies** If you're planning to get pregnant in the near future, or discover you are pregnant while taking any medication (long or short term), speak to a healthcare professional about your current medications or supplements routine. Some medicines, treatments and remedies are safe to take in pregnancy, but some can be potentially harmful to a developing baby. They'll advise if you should continue using your medication, adapt the dosage, switch to something else, or stop altogether.[9]
- **Stop smoking and vaping** Smoking, and being around passive smoking, can affect fertility, so it's recommended to

quit before trying for a baby. After conceiving, smoking in pregnancy, and being around other people who smoke, can be very harmful for a developing baby. It has been linked with higher rates of miscarriage and developmental problems, as well as low birth weight (which can lead to further complications). Stopping smoking also reduces the risk of sudden infant death syndrome (SIDS), also known as cot death. There is a complete lack of evidence about vaping, so fertility experts recommend stopping vaping too. Quitting smoking can be incredibly challenging, but there is support out there to help you (see Resources).

- **Limit alcohol** Drinking alcohol is also linked to fertility problems, and alcohol can be harmful in early pregnancy. If you're trying to conceive, the safest advice is to try to avoid alcohol altogether.
- **'Healthy' weight** We've already touched on BMI in Chapter 6, and why it's a flawed system of measuring how 'healthy' or 'unhealthy' a person is. However, as all medical guidelines use it, your GP will likely include it in their watch-outs list for trying to conceive, especially if you're trying to access fertility treatments. Generally, aiming for a BMI between 18.5 and 25 may help your chances of conceiving and having a healthy pregnancy. Having a BMI over 30 is associated with a longer time to conceive, reduced rates of conceiving and also reduced responsiveness to fertility treatments. And in some areas, if your BMI is over 30 you may not be able to access fertility treatments on the NHS. Lowering your BMI will also reduce your risk of complications during pregnancy and delivery.
- **Exercise** We all know that exercise is good for us, but it can really help when trying for a baby. Being physically active can improve your fertility and boost chances of conceiving, as well as improving the chances of a healthy pregnancy with

fewer complications. At least 150 minutes of moderate aerobic activity a week and strength exercises on two or more days a week can make a difference. Be mindful of avoiding excessive exercise, which can stress the body into not ovulating.

- **A balanced diet** Becoming more conscious of what you're eating will help ensure you're getting varied, nutrient-rich foods, which is key when it comes to trying to conceive and throughout pregnancy. There is evidence to suggest that the Mediterranean-style diet – so eating lots of fruit, veg, wholegrains, oily fish and lean proteins – may be protective against infertility.[10] If you're vegan or vegetarian, you might find it more difficult to get enough iron and vitamin B12. So if you're vegan or vegetarian, or you follow a restricted diet because of food intolerance (for example, a gluten-free diet for coeliac disease) or for religious reasons, consider speaking to a dietitian.
- **Cervical screenings** Ensuring you're up to date with your cervical screening is really important. Anyone with a cervix between the ages of twenty-five and sixty-four should be having these routinely to test for human papillomavirus (HPV), a very common virus, some strains of which can cause changes to the cells in the cervix that can, over time, cause cervical cancer. Cervical screening is usually avoided during pregnancy or for twelve weeks after delivery, so if you're not up to date it's a good idea to go for a test before trying to conceive. Lots of fertility services also ask for an up-to-date cervical screening test before you can be referred.
- **Hydration** 'Drink more water' – we're sure you've heard that time and time again – but it's important to note that keeping hydrated can actually improve your cervical fluid around ovulation, which can help sperm reach an egg.
- **Caffeine** When it comes to caffeine, there isn't a clear link to show whether it affects fertility, but research has

shown that drinking a lot of coffee, tea and caffeinated soft drinks may increase the time it takes to get pregnant and may affect the health of a developing baby.[11] So if you are pregnant or trying to conceive, it's recommended that you limit your daily caffeine intake to 200 milligrams per day (approximately two cups of coffee, but this can vary).

*Sperm optimisation (now there's a phrase)*

There is so much focus on the female anatomy when it comes to trying to get pregnant, but of course, there's often another person involved. Various factors can affect male fertility, including issues like having a low sperm count, low-quality sperm and/or motility problems (i.e. how effective sperm is at travelling to fertilise an egg).

- **Drugs and stimulants** Did you know that smoking, drinking in excess of recommended limits and recreational drug use – including cannabis and anabolic steroids – can reduce sperm quality?[12] There are plenty of ways a partner or donor can help maximise the chance of pregnancy,[13] and not cutting these vices out or drinking within recommended limits could make conceiving more difficult.
- **Environmental factors** Exposure to certain pesticides, solvents and metals has been shown to affect fertility, particularly in men.[14] Synthetic chemicals, such as Bisphenol-A (BPA) found in plastics, and phthalates and parabens found in beauty and cleaning products, are known as 'endocrine disruptors', meaning they can affect hormones and may impact your fertility, although more research is needed into this.[15] Reducing exposure to these and choosing paraben-free alternatives is often recommended by fertility experts.
- **Sperm quality** This can be affected by temperature. Studies have shown that using hot tubs or even hot baths can impair fertility (only slightly, mind) but luckily using

your laptop on your knee, saunas or those lovely heated car seats seem to be OK.[16] Sports such as cycling can cause sperm concentration, mobility and number to decrease – but we're unsure if this is due to temperature, or just pure saddle trauma.[17]

- **The big five** You guessed it – a balanced, nutritious diet; having a 'healthy' BMI; keeping fit; lowering stress and stopping smoking are all recommended for high-quality sperm. Although stress is an interesting one . . .

*Can stress impact fertility?*

Here we brought in the help of our expert fertility nurse consultant Kate Davies. Kate is the ultimate fountain of knowledge on all things fertility and has supported hundreds of people to conceive, both through her private clinic and via her super popular podcast – The Fertility Podcast.

'Contrary to popular belief, there is no evidence to suggest that stress ITSELF impacts on reproductive outcomes BUT it is what we do as a result of stress that does have an impact, such as hitting the bottle, smoking to help stress relief, making poor nutritional choices, not getting enough sleep etc. However, we do know that problems conceiving equals stress and therefore working on strategies to help manage stress and seeking professional help can make all the difference.'

**Keep them cool**

Over to Kate again. We asked her opinion on spa days and bicycles . . .

'Although the impact of a hot bath or lounging in the hot tub or sauna may be minimal, it is certainly something we would recommend avoiding as a man when you are actively trying to conceive. At this stage you want to do everything you can to increase your chances and avoiding a hot bath, hot tub or sauna is probably a change that is reasonably easy to do for the short term. As we're unsure about the impact of cycling on sperm health, I advise my patients to avoid cycling for long periods of time (a short cycle to work is fine), as the length of time in lycra equals hotter testicles, which in turn impacts on sperm production. A man's testicles are outside the body for a very good reason, they need to be kept at a lower temperature than body temperature, but can heat up quickly in lycra! And it looks like that uncomfortable little seat on a man's bike has a part to play too!'

There are conditions which can permanently impact a male's ability to make healthy sperm, such as viruses like mumps or previous cancer treatment. To find out what's happening with your partner's sperm, their GP will refer them for a semen analysis. This is where your partner has to provide a sample into a pot (often not their most enjoyable solo experience) and the sperm is inspected under a microscope. If problems are identified, a fertility clinic will be needed to provide support and advice.

**Fertility experience**
Trying for 1–3 years   29 years old

My partner and I have been trying to conceive for about a year and three months now. It's so hard. I never thought it would affect me as much as it has. We have only just been referred to the 'infertility' clinic locally, but they're unable to advise wait times. My partner's sperm count was not just low but also a few other things, which can change with his diet, which he has/is doing. I've been told the classic – get your BMI to X,Y,Z. I'm about a size 14. I struggle with friends' baby announcements, but I am so so happy for them, it just hurts it's not me. I hate how others feel it's OK to ask when you're having your kids etc. I have some great days when I feel fine then I have days/weeks where all I do is cry. I feel there's so little support and help, despite how common the difficulties of getting pregnant are. I was on the contraceptive pill for years. And I had a [miscarriage] at about seventeen years old and a termination in my early twenties. I find myself thinking what if so often. I'm hoping that I'm not the only one who has such ups and downs and struggles. I just want it to [be] my turn for a little family now. Finding this forum, I am hoping makes me feel more human. Thank you for reading in advance.

Shared on **thelowdown.com**

## When's best to take a pregnancy test?

Ah, the two-week wait. This is the two weeks between ovulation and when you'll either get a positive pregnancy result on a test or get your period. This can feel like a hellishly long time full of anticipation, excitement or anxiety, whether you desperately want that positive result or very much do not.

The timing of taking a pregnancy test matters – too early and it can lead to a false negative. It really is best to wait at least fourteen days after ovulation or the day after your period is due to take a test, and some people advise you to take it in the morning when your urine is most concentrated. This allows time for the pregnancy hormone hCG (human chorionic gonadotrophin) to be raised enough to show on a home-testing kit. It can be a stressful time – especially if you have been trying to conceive for a while and/or you have suffered pregnancy loss in the past. Look after yourself, pull out all the stops for some self-care and avoid doing anything you wouldn't do in early pregnancy (so, no smoking or alcohol).

## What if you're *not* getting pregnant?

It's important to acknowledge that you can do everything we've listed previously, have no obvious underlying conditions, and still have trouble getting (or staying) pregnant. Similarly, there are lots of people who don't do things by the book and get pregnant easily. The world can be chaotic, unpredictable and unfair.

We know it's normal to take up to a year to conceive naturally. This could be down to a number of factors. Age, genetics, general health as well as any underlying medical conditions influence our fertility. And, infertility issues are common, with one in six people worldwide being affected.[18] If you're not getting pregnant within twelve months, or within six months if you're over thirty-five or have a known reproductive health condition like PCOS or endometriosis, make an appointment to see your GP to ask for a referral to a fertility clinic.

**What will a GP do if I'm not getting pregnant?**

For referral to an NHS fertility clinic, your GP will need to make sure you fulfil the local NHS criteria and start some initial tests. These may include:

- Basic information about you and your partner's age, BMI, medical history and pregnancy histories.
- Hormonal blood tests taken at the start of your cycle (oestrogen, FSH and LH levels) and seven days before your next predicted period, usually on day twenty-one (progesterone levels). If you don't have periods, you may be prescribed progestogen tablets to cause a bleed.
- Blood test screening to check your immunity to Rubella, a virus which can affect a growing pregnancy (you will be offered vaccination before fertility treatment if you're not immune).
- Cervical screening if it's not up to date.
- An STI screen.
- Semen analysis if you have a male partner.

---

**Q:** Are there any hormone tests I can do to check my fertility?

**A:** One type of fertility hormone test that's used is anti-müllerian hormone (AMH) testing. AMH is produced by the follicles (small sacs on the ovaries) that contain immature eggs. Because of this, AMH blood testing is sometimes used as a marker for fertility by estimating how many eggs you have left in your ovaries, known as your ovarian reserve.

However, AMH should not be used alone as a marker of fertility. AMH levels are affected by age, BMI and hormonal

**Fertility experience**
Trying for 1-3 years 29 years old

When we first started trying, I really thought we would get pregnant straightaway. My husband has a daughter already and no-one in our family has ever struggled before, so why wouldn't we, right? Well as the months went by, it got harder and harder to survive the two-week wait and see test after test be negative. By this point, three of my closest friends all got pregnant and now, fourteen months later, they're all expecting and I haven't even managed to get pregnant yet. It feels so isolating and like you're the only person in the world going through it. I have tried joining some forums and groups but they seem to be plagued with pictures and stories of babies and less focused on the people who haven't got to that stage yet. All in all, it does make you feel like giving up. We're now at the stage of getting tests done to see if there is anything we can do medically to help, but I do feel like there isn't enough support out there for those of us on our journey.

Shared on **thelowdown.com**

contraception, especially the combined pill. AMH testing was also developed to help inform IVF treatment and not as a predictor of natural fertility or egg quality. So while lower levels are indicative of lower ovarian reserve, many people will conceive without problems. On the other hand, others with an AMH level indicating a good ovarian reserve may take time to conceive and need fertility treatment.[19] Tests for AMH can be purchased privately, but this can cause more harm than good if the results aren't explained in your individual context by healthcare professionals. All other hormone tests are available from your GP. However, if you are having regular periods with a normal cycle length, these tests are unlikely to add anything and are only relevant if you are struggling to conceive.

## Looking after your mental health

If having a baby is taking longer than you'd anticipated, it can really take its toll on your mental health. It doesn't help if you've reached a certain age and it suddenly seems like everyone you know is expecting. Well-meaning (read: annoying) people ask when you're going to hurry up and have a baby or blithely offer unsolicited comments on your family planning. It can be rough, and it's a time shrouded in a lot of mystery – no one talks about how isolating it can feel. Whatever stage you're at on your fertility journey, the upcoming advice is also worth trying.

- **Reducing stress** Yes, it's easier said than done. If you've decided to try for a baby, or have been trying for longer than you thought you would be, it can be stressful and exhausting. It's easy to become fixated on the calendar, diligently scheduling sex. 'Trying mode' can be all-consuming. It can become even more of a pressure cooker if you suffer from conditions which can (for some people) make getting pregnant more difficult, such as endometriosis or PCOS, which we'll come on to. Focus on ways that make you feel relaxed and take the strain out of organised sex. Some couples find boosting intimacy in other ways helps them feel more connected and less hassled by the process. Spending time together doing something you both like is a good place to start.
- **Talk about it** Talking about fertility stress with someone you trust can be so helpful. If you're talking to your partner,

you might find you're both feeling the same. Deciding to take baby-talk off the table for a bit to reconnect, before revisiting it, could help. If you're talking to friends or family, you'll most likely be surprised at how many others go through these things too. We'd suggest setting some boundaries for the conversation before you begin if you're not looking for advice, just a listening ear. Saying, 'Things are tough right now, I don't need advice, just some support', can really make all the difference. Letting your loved ones know that you've started trying could also help them understand any changes in your behaviour, and provide a much-needed support network.

The more we talk about pregnancy loss, fertility struggles and fertility treatment, the more we normalise these topics being spoken about out in the open. On page 364 in the Resources, we list some great organisations that offer support for people going through fertility problems, including advice on how to navigate discussing it at work or telling family members.

## Conditions that can impact fertility

It's not always possible for doctors to get to the root cause of fertility issues, as sometimes tests reveal inconclusive results. Other times, the causes are more obvious, which can be helpful as it means medical teams can have a targeted approach to fertility treatment. A more personalised approach to fertility (and all aspects of our health) is something we'd love to see more of in future.

In Chapter 4, we looked at polycystic ovary syndrome (PCOS) and endometriosis. Let's delve into them again here as they can sometimes have an impact on getting pregnant.

## Fertility and PCOS

PCOS affects the ability to ovulate, which is essential for pregnancy to happen. The hormonal imbalance associated with PCOS means ovulation may not happen (anovulation) or may be unpredictable. Irregular or absent periods are a sign that ovulation might not be happening regularly, or at all. On top of this, anyone with irregular periods will attest it's really difficult to work out your fertile days and when to have sex to maximise the chances of pregnancy.

> **Fertility experience**
> Trying for 1-3 years   35 years old
>
> We came off the pill and started trying for around a year. I have PCOS so I knew it wouldn't be easy. I fell pregnant but had a missed miscarriage around seven weeks. It then took about three years before we conceived our daughter.
>
> Shared on **thelowdown.com**

*Improving fertility*

If PCOS affects your fertility, it can be incredibly draining. While you feel ready for a baby, your body hasn't quite got the memo. As we've looked at on pages 113–4, lifestyle changes can play a huge role in easing PCOS symptoms, and the list of tips on pages 260–7 to improve your fertility are all still relevant if you have PCOS. International guidelines state that lifestyle changes are the first-line option to treat fertility issues relating to PCOS. There are lots of actions you can take yourself without involvement from a healthcare professional, such as reducing your intake of refined carbs (i.e. sugary, processed carbs) and starting strength training. But many find it helpful to get support from a dietitian or nutritionist specialising in PCOS, as if you are overweight losing just 5 per cent of your body weight can have a really positive impact on your fertility by restoring regular periods and ovulation while also improving pregnancy outcomes.[20]

A popular supplement called myo-inositol has been shown to improve ovulation in some people with PCOS.[21] The research to support myo-inositol isn't brilliant, but it's a very safe supplement so is unlikely to do any harm to try, as it may help. If you choose to take myo-inositol, another supplement called alpha-lactalbumin can help your body absorb more of the myo-inositol, possibly making it more effective.[22] These supplements can be expensive and you should speak to a healthcare professional before using them, especially if you're taking any other medication.

*What if you have PCOS and are not getting pregnant?*

There are a number of possible reasons this may be the case, aside from PCOS, including your partner having fertility issues. Also, as covered on page 250, if you've recently come off contraception, it can take a few months for your cycle to return to what is normal for you, which can be a reason for the delay. However, you should be referred for fertility support after six months of trying to conceive if you have PCOS.

There are plenty of options out there to help with PCOS-related fertility problems, which are often successful. Some women find digital ovulation predictors, such as OvuSense, helpful. This is a vaginal sensor which tracks your core body temperature in order to help predict when you're about to ovulate. Some find methods like this more effective than other ways to cycle-track or urine ovulation predictor sticks. In PCOS, the lack of ovulation is often the cause of issues. Medication can be used to induce ovulation, or there are treatments such as IVF.

### Fertility and endometriosis

As we saw in Chapter 4, endometriosis is a condition where cells similar to those in the uterus are found in other parts of the body. Like PCOS, it can affect your quality of life. Endometriosis, what causes it and how it progresses, aren't fully understood yet but we know it can impact the reproductive organs, including the ovaries and fallopian tubes. It can cause scar tissue where pelvic organs become stuck together through inflammation or ovarian cysts. Up to 50 per cent of women undergoing fertility tests or treatment are found to have endometriosis and for many of them, struggling to get pregnant is their only symptom.[23]

Again, our previous list of tips to improve your fertility still applies if you have endometriosis. If you want further intervention, surgical removal of endometrial deposits and cysts is a treatment option which has been shown to improve fertility and help manage pain.[24] If you opt for surgery, the best time to try to conceive with endometriosis is thought to be soon after having the deposits or cysts removed. There is no evidence other drug treatments for endometriosis improve fertility.

#### *How long will it take to get pregnant?*

Of those couples trying to conceive naturally where endometriosis is a factor, most (60–70 per cent) will get pregnant within one year of trying, compared to over 80 per cent of couples where endometriosis is not an issue.[25] As we've ascertained, everyone is different and there's unfortunately no concrete answer when it comes to how long it can take to get pregnant.

One endometriosis fertility factor seems to be related to the severity of endometriosis found through laparoscopic surgery – 75 per cent of women with mild, 50 per cent with moderate and 25 per cent with severe endometriosis will conceive within one year of trying.[26] Nothing is set in stone, of course, and even those with severe symptoms can become pregnant in the first month of trying.

> **Fertility experience**
> Trying for 6 months    30 years old
>
> I had my Mirena coil removed and switched to Natural Cycles about three months before trying to conceive. It then only took two months of trying before falling pregnant, which really surprised me as I have endometriosis and only one functioning ovary, so I feel very lucky it was so easy for us. Natural Cycles was so helpful for knowing when I was ovulating and understanding my cycle much better. I also use ovulation tests on the second month of trying, which, once you get the hang of them, were good too. The intimacy side is quite odd – we really went hard at trying when I was ovulating, so we had to put in a lot of effort to keep it fun and interesting.
>
> Shared on **thelowdown.com**

*What if you have endometriosis and are not getting pregnant?*

As we've seen, it's totally normal for it to take up to a year to get pregnant even without conditions like endometriosis or PCOS. However, if you're diagnosed with endometriosis, you may be able to get referred for fertility support and treatment earlier than those who don't have it. Depending on where you are in the world, this may include further tests and support to get pregnant if you haven't conceived within six months of trying. Speak to your GP about what's available in your area.

There may also be private options if means allow, which may have shorter waiting lists.

Fertility specialists may offer surgery to remove or treat deposits or cysts or suggest fertility treatments like ovulation induction or IVF. If the stress of trying to conceive is getting to you, and you'd like more support with dealing with endometriosis' symptoms while going through it, check out our Resources.

### Other conditions that can affect fertility

Similarly to PCOS, conditions that affect your ability to ovulate can impair your fertility. Thyroid problems (both under- or overactive thyroid) may mean you may struggle to release eggs. Premature ovarian insufficiency (also known as premature menopause) is where your ovaries stop functioning normally before the age of forty, meaning ovulation stops or happens infrequently.

Other illnesses and conditions can affect your ability to get pregnant. Diabetes and autoimmune problems are common culprits. Not only that, but these conditions need to be well managed to make sure a pregnancy can grow and develop well. Many people may benefit from a referral for preconception counselling from a specialist medical team. For example, women with diabetes will have strict glucose targets to try to achieve before getting pregnant. These conversations are important so you understand what you can do to optimise your condition and manage symptoms to boost your fertility and the chances of a healthy pregnancy.

Pelvic inflammatory disease (PID) can be caused by an untreated infection or STI. This can cause scarring in the fallopian tubes which prevents an egg travelling down from the ovary to meet sperm. This unfortunately leads to fertility problems in around 18 per cent of those with PID.[27]

Fibroids are common but often not mentioned as a cause of fertility issues; however, depending on where they are, they can prevent a fertilised egg from implanting into the uterus lining, or even block a fallopian tube.

Finally, we shouldn't forget the rarer conditions that some women are born with that affect the ability to conceive or carry a child, or those who have undergone cancer treatment. As we mentioned at the beginning of this chapter, there are many routes to starting a family if it's something you want.

## Assisted conception and fertility treatments

If you've been trying and things just aren't happening naturally, fertility clinics are here to help.

### What investigations will a fertility clinic do?

Over again to Independent Fertility Nurse Consultant, Kate Davies: 'Once you've been referred to the fertility clinic, it is likely that your specialist will want to do some further tests. This might include blood tests, a sperm test (if not already done and if you have a male partner) and scans to look at your uterus and ovaries. You may be offered a procedure to look at your fallopian tubes (basically to make sure these important little structures are not blocked). This investigation may be called a HyCosy or HSG. It's not the most pleasant test and may cause discomfort but it's over really quickly and you only need to have it done once. Other tests and investigations may be recommended if you have, or might have, any conditions impacting on your fertility such as investigating endometriosis, PCOS, uterine abnormalities or if you have sadly suffered from pregnancy loss in the past.'

There are several potential fertility treatments that can be used. Some of these assisted conception methods are relatively low intervention, like taking medications such as letrozole, clomiphene or metformin to induce ovulation (especially in PCOS).

Assisted conception can, however, get even more sophisticated. You might have assisted conception if fertility issues mean you've struggled to become pregnant or maintain a pregnancy. It might also be used if you're unable to have vaginal sex, are a same-sex couple or a single person wanting to become a parent. We so often hear from Lowdown users that they wish they'd known more about assisted conception before starting their journey, so let's get into it.

There are three main types:

- Intrauterine insemination (IUI)
- In vitro fertilisation (IVF)
- Intracytoplasmic sperm injection (ICSI)

• **IUI** is when sperm is injected into the uterus at the time of ovulation. This can either be done during a natural cycle, where the female partner ovulates naturally, or by using fertility medications to stimulate ovulation. The sperm is washed and filtered to identify the top swimmers and then injected into the uterus. This is a more common option for same-sex female couples.

• **IVF** is a medical procedure that's been used around the world since the late 1970s.[28] Eggs are removed from the body, mixed with sperm 'in vitro', i.e. in a lab, grown for a few days then inserted into the uterus. It sounds simple but it is *actually* incredible and the treatment plan requires a lot of medical finesse to make it individualised, and good time organisation from the people undergoing treatment.

The process of IVF can differ a little depending on the clinic you attend and/or your medical situation. Most of the time, the first stage involves suppressing your menstrual cycle. You then take medication for ten to fourteen days to stimulate egg growth in the ovaries. This helps you develop more mature eggs than you ordinarily would in your regular menstrual cycle, and you'll be monitored during this time by the clinic to see how you're responding to the medication. In a minor surgical procedure, under sedation, your eggs will then be removed. At this point, eggs can be frozen (which is known as oocyte cryopreservation) or they can be combined with sperm (which can be from a partner or a donor). Once the eggs and sperm fertilise, they become embryos. These embryos are then left for around five days in a lab to develop. You'll be given hormone medication to help your uterus get ready for what's called the 'embryo transfer'. This is when one or two of the best-quality embryos will be transferred back into the uterus, while any remaining embryos can be frozen for possible future use. The embryo transfer procedure is less invasive than the egg removal stage, and you most likely won't need sedation. The embryo is then left to its own devices, hopefully implanting into the uterus lining. If it has been successful, you'll have a positive pregnancy test two weeks later.

- **ICSI** follows the same process as IVF, but rather than mixing sperm with the eggs, a single sperm is isolated and injected directly into the egg – amazing, right?

Unfortunately, assisted conception isn't always guaranteed to work, even after several rounds. There can be some trial and error if you decide on subsequent attempts, where your medical team can refine their approach based on how your body responds to the treatment. This can take a physical and emotional toll, which we know lots of people don't always feel prepared for.

**Fertility experience**
Trying for 1–3 years 34 years old

The experience was stressful! Being told to have fun trying by well-meaning friends – anyone who has had problems conceiving knows it's not fun! Emotions run high and it felt very lonely, as I didn't want to make people feel awkward or uncomfortable by giving them the honest answer when they asked if we wanted to have children. I used ovulation kits and tracking apps but it's easy to become obsessive about dates and numbers. In the end we had IVF and got pregnant on the first round. Now our baby boy is three months old.

Shared on **thelowdown.com**

If you're resident in the UK seeking to become pregnant through methods such as IVF, your doctor will assess your potential suitability and you may be able to access treatment through the NHS. This rests on certain criteria being met, such as medical suitability and history, age and lifestyle factors, how long you've been trying to get pregnant through unprotected sex (if this applies to you), and whether or not you have other children.

Unfortunately, it can also be a bit of a 'postcode lottery' with some parts of the country better provided for than others. For 'unexplained fertility' (where no obvious reason is identified to be causing infertility, such as an underlying medical condition) the NICE (National Institute for Health and Care Excellence) guideline suggests that women in the UK who have been trying unsuccessfully to conceive for two years should be offered IVF.[29] Otherwise, there are private options available, though they can be expensive. We're also seeing some clinics only charge for IVF if treatment has been successful.

## Fertility treatment inequality

Seeking fertility treatments like IVF has been on the rise since 2020,[30] but despite this rise there are still lots of barriers in place. A survey by The Fawcett Society of 2,000 people found that one in five undergoing fertility treatment quit their jobs because they were treated poorly at work by their colleagues or management.[31] This is alongside the obvious barrier of the physical and mental strain that going through these types of treatments can put you under.

On top of all of that, the financial strain that may come with accessing treatments can also be demanding. This is even more of an issue if you're in a same-sex couple, or trying to go through treatment as a single person, or come from an underprivileged socio-economic or ethnic minority background. Historically, female same-sex couples have had to fund multiple rounds of IVF themselves before being able to access NHS services.[32] For many years, an outdated UK law required same-sex couples to pay up to £1,000 for safety screening for infectious diseases, while heterosexual couples have not had to pay for this. This legislation has thankfully been axed.[33]

Black, Asian and minority ethnic women are also drastically impacted by fertility inequality, as shown in a 2021 report by the Human Fertilisation and Embryology Authority (the UK's fertility regulator), which stated that Black women are twenty-five times less likely to access fertility treatment at all.[34] Health outcomes for these women are shamefully poorer overall across the country, and when it comes to accessing fertility treatment, this report also showed they have 7 per cent less chance of having a baby than white women.[35] This is down to factors like struggling to find access to sperm donors from similar backgrounds, cultural and religious barriers, and the fact that lots of fertility treatment advertising is aimed at white women.

# 10

# Contraception after pregnancy

If you've just given birth, the only thing you may want to do between the sheets is ... sleep. On the other hand, you might feel relieved not to have a baby bump getting in the way and are raring to go all over again. Whichever camp you fall into (and maybe it's a bit of both, energy-depending!), it's a good idea to make a plan when it comes to your contraceptive options. It may not be high on the priorities list when you're busy buying nappies and cleaning baby sick out of your hair, but your GP will likely raise your contraceptive options in your routine six-to-eight-week postpartum appointment. So with this in mind, it can make sense to think about future contraceptive options *before* your baby arrives and the sleepless nights take hold. If you're in a relationship, you might like to include your partner in discussions about this.

So, in this chapter, we look at your post-baby contraceptive options, those that are safe while breastfeeding, whether breastfeeding is a reliable contraceptive in itself, and how soon you can start different methods. We'll also look at how your contraceptive needs may have changed now that there's an infant on the scene (who, let's face it, is probably getting in the way of your sex life), and why your previous contraceptive method, which may have worked well for you pre-baby, just isn't hitting the same.

## Sex after pregnancy and birth

There are no guidelines on how long you need to wait after giving birth before you can have sex, so do what feels right for you. However, if you have had a complicated birth that involved the use of instruments, stitches, a Caesarean section (C-section) or a post-op infection, you might like to wait until you're healed or have had a chance to discuss sex at your six-to-eight-week postpartum review. You're likely to be pretty sore as your body will need to recover from growing a new human for nine months; giving birth, vaginally or via C-section, puts your body through extremes. Understandably, you and your partner might feel nervous about postpartum sex – particularly if you've had stitches, as the area will be tender and vulnerable to pressure. Post-pregnancy hormones and a drop in oestrogen, especially if you are breastfeeding, can cause vaginal dryness. So take it easy, lube up, and stop if it's too painful. If your body's not back to feeling 100 per cent, but your sex drive is, you can always take penetrative sex off the table while you recover.

But it's not all changes to *your* libido; partners may feel this too. Plus, there's the small matter of exhaustion to contend with. The carousel of feeding, changing nappies, getting babies to sleep and soothing them through discomfort doesn't stop. If you're breastfeeding, these hormones may reduce your sex drive, which could be seen as nature's way of natural child spacing.

## How soon can you get pregnant again after giving birth?

There's a range of what's considered 'normal' when it comes to postpartum fertility. It's possible to get pregnant from having sex as soon as twenty-one days after you give birth, and it's impossible to predict exactly when your fertility will return.

Some people have their first period around six or so weeks after giving birth, while for others it can take months, even years, to return. It varies from person to person as a result of physiological differences as well as individual hormonal make-up. And how you choose to feed your baby plays a significant part, as most women (though not all!) who exclusively breastfeed will have a delay in their cycle returning, so might fit the criteria to use breastfeeding as a contraceptive (yes, really), which we'll dive into later in the chapter.

When your periods do return, they can initially feel different to how they were before getting pregnant. Changes might be related to how long or short they are, how heavy or light the flow is and any other symptoms you experience. Many women report periods being more of a handful for the first few cycles, with heavier or longer bleeding. They can also keep you on your toes by arriving and then disappearing again, taking a while to settle into any kind of rhythm. It can be the case that while your period has returned, you may not be ovulating each cycle and you won't necessarily be able to tell if you are or not (see page 22 for more on anovulatory cycles). This is simply because your body is adjusting to the new balance of hormones.

## Why bother thinking about contraception?

Given it's possible to get pregnant from three weeks after giving birth, it's not uncommon for someone to be caught out with an unplanned pregnancy, having not even realised their fertility had returned. This is sometimes called 'catching the first egg' because ovulation happens *before* the fertility warning signal of the first period. So, you can go from one pregnancy to the next without having a period in-between. Some people may be thrilled with the prospect of being pregnant again so soon, though for many others, it may come as a blow and tough decisions will have to be made.

The World Health Organization recommends leaving a minimum of eighteen months, but preferably twenty-four months, between pregnancies, to help ensure the healthiest outcomes for mother and baby. This is particularly important for women in low- to middle-income countries, but a large study from Canada found that a twelve-month gap between pregnancies was similar in risk to an eighteen- to twenty-four-month gap. So for women in the UK, a twelve-month gap may be more applicable.[1] If you've had a C-section, it's advised to wait at least twelve months to allow your uterus to fully heal before getting pregnant. Having a gap between pregnancies is, of course, an individual choice, and people in their mid-to-late thirties or older may be weighing up the risk of a short time between pregnancies alongside the risk of fertility issues as they get older. Contraception can put you in the driving seat of your fertility, helping you to choose if and when you decide to try for another baby.

---

**Q:** I used the progestogen-only pill before coming off to conceive. I experienced some annoying side effects from it but generally felt OK. If I start using it again post-pregnancy, will I feel the same?

**A:** Many of us wonder if our side effects on a certain contraceptive will change after we've had a baby. Unfortunately, as with much of women's health, this hasn't been researched extensively (surprise, surprise). There has been some patchy research on bleeding patterns with the implant and injection after pregnancy. Two studies have shown that the bleeding pattern expected with the injection postpartum is no different to bleeding patterns if a woman uses the injection before pregnancy, but these were not high-quality studies.[2] Several studies have shown that the discontinuation rate for all women using the implant due to bleeding problems is 16–20 per cent,[3] and this is reflected similarly for women after pregnancy, where the discontinuation rate due to bleeding problems is 18–21 per cent.[4] The timing of starting the implant after delivery also makes no difference to change in bleeding pattern.[5] Annoyingly, there is no research on more complex side effects such as mood change. Anecdotally, though, we have heard stories from Lowdown users who have been really settled on a method of contraception before they got pregnant. On returning to the same method after pregnancy, they found their side effects were completely different! We believe this is only a small minority of people, so you may well not experience much, if any, difference if you do go back to your previous method. As ever, we would love to see more research carried out in this area.

---

Here's the experience of one Lowdown user who, after they'd given birth, was put on the same type of pill, although a different brand, but had a wildly different experience.

**Progestogen-only/mini pill**
Used for 1–3 months   No age shared

★☆☆☆☆

**Cerelle pill**

I was on the Cerazette pill for about five years before falling pregnant and had no problems whatsoever. After I had my baby, I went to the doctors to be placed back on the same pill, but I was told they no longer prescribe Cerazette and have replaced it with Cerelle. I was on this pill for six weeks before I had to take myself off it. My mood swings were horrendous – I was crying most days over silly little things! I couldn't stand my partner and I always thought he wasn't doing anything for me and the baby. I've been off Cerelle for a week now, and my whole life has done a complete U turn. I'm back to my happy loving self, I cannot get enough of my partner and I realise now he goes to the ends of the earth for me and his son. Now to find another one that actually works!

Shared on **thelowdown.com**

## Breastfeeding as a form of contraception

The lactational amenorrhea method (LAM) refers to using breastfeeding as a contraceptive method. Yep, it's a thing. LAM relies on the hormones that stimulate breastfeeding to prevent ovulation, and in turn, pause your fertility. This is a hotly debated topic whenever we mention it on The Lowdown. As with other fertility awareness methods (FAM), some people use it successfully and love it, while others find that they've ended up unexpectedly pregnant. Which, when you've had a baby within the last year, isn't often the top of your priority list. If used correctly, LAM is around 98 per cent effective. The criteria for using breastfeeding as an effective method must be closely followed to ensure it works; it's a method where there's easily room for human error. Hello, new-parent sleep deprivation.

Here's what you need to know. The main three criteria for LAM are:

- Your baby is less than six months old.
- You are exclusively breastfeeding day and night, i.e. you haven't used any formula.
- Your periods have not returned.

'Exclusive' breastfeeding in this sense means not feeding them any formula or food and you are feeding responsively as your baby wants milk (rather than following a set schedule). It also means feeding from the breast as opposed to expressing your milk. Many parents find the more frequently their baby exclusively breastfeeds, the longer the delay to their fertility returning.

If you are breastfeeding exclusively 'on demand' (aka 'responsive feeding'), at least every four hours in the day and every six hours at night, your periods haven't returned and your baby is under six months old, you are unlikely to be fertile. But breastfeeding is hard, and the hands-on support available depends on where you live, which is why we're lucky to have the option of formula or combination feeding. If you want to breastfeed, we have included some fantastic organisations who can help in the Resources. In the UK, where breastfeeding rates are very low versus other countries, only 24 per cent of mothers are exclusively breastfeeding by the time their baby is six weeks old; by six months old, this has dropped to around 1 per cent.[6]

If you're going to try out LAM as a contraceptive after giving birth, even just one of the following factors will reduce its effectiveness:

- Your baby breastfeeding less frequently and having longer gaps between feeds (like if you are separated or if your baby starts to sleep longer through the night).
- If you're expressing milk.
- The introduction of formula, juice or solids.
- Using a dummy or comforter.
- Illness, stress or anxiety with either you or the baby.

If any of these circumstances change, an alternative – and more reliable – form of contraception will be needed if you're not looking to get pregnant again almost straight away after giving birth.

Some people can tell if their periods are going to make a reappearance soon thanks to telltale signs in the weeks before, such as PMS symptoms or changes to their cervical fluid. If you are attuned to these signals, it's very much time to use contraception if you're not planning on pregnancy any time soon. If you no longer meet the LAM criteria or just want other options, the good news is there are plenty of safe options available while breastfeeding, so let's get into it.

## Contraception after birth

So, you've got your twenty-one-day grace period after giving birth, where you can't get pregnant. Even so, you might want to start a method before this window closes to ensure you're covered.

### What can you start straight away?

Some contraception can be started immediately after birth, which takes the hassle away from having to think about it later on. Your options include progestogen-only contraceptives as well as the copper coil (which is non-hormonal). These are all safe to use while breastfeeding:

- Progestogen-only pill.
- Injection.
- Implant.
- Hormonal coil (IUS).
- Copper coil.

If you're in the UK, ideally, maternity services should always be able to offer you a contraceptive injection, implant or coil immediately after birth. However, unfortunately, in reality this might not always be possible due to staffing and the timing of your delivery. If that's the case, you should be signposted to where you can get your chosen contraceptive and provided with an alternative in the meantime.

### When can you start combined contraception?

Combined hormonal contraception (the pill, ring or patch) can be safely started six weeks after giving birth if you're medically eligible to use it, whether you are breastfeeding or not. If you aren't breastfeeding, you may be able to start combined contraception after three weeks as long as you have no other risk factors for blood clots like smoking, a raised BMI or have had a C-section (as surgical procedures and the lack of mobility following them also increase the risk of blood clots – hence why you have to wear those horrible long socks . . .).

The longer delay before you can start combined contraception is all because of blood clot risk (see page 192). During pregnancy and the six-week period just after giving birth, you have a higher risk of blood clots, which is greater than taking any type or brand of combined contraception. The chance of you having a blood clot increases with the addition of each separate risk factor, with the postpartum period being a major one.

### *Hormonal contraception and breastfeeding*

Current research shows that progestogen-only contraceptive methods do not affect milk supply or your baby's growth or development. While this research is clear, the information for the combined hormonal pill is less so, with concerns that the oestrogen within combined methods may reduce supply – especially if started within six weeks after delivery.[7]

There have been extensive reviews examining these studies into breast milk supply, which determine that the research isn't high enough quality and may have been affected by data from women who were using old-fashioned types and doses of the combined pill. However, we're confident that the research into baby's growth and development is better quality, and shows that infant outcomes aren't affected by the combined pill when compared with the progestogen-only pill[8] – so if your baby is more than six weeks old and it's your number-one choice while breastfeeding and safe for you, then go ahead. If you are concerned about dips in your supply, there are often ways to boost it – in our Resources (page 362) we list organisations that can support you with breastfeeding.

## Barrier methods

Both male and female condoms can be used straight after delivery. If you use a diaphragm, you'll need to wait for six weeks after delivery for the uterus to shrink back down and, as your size may have changed, you'll need to have another fitting. It's advisable to use another method in the meantime.

## Fertility awareness methods (FAM)

FAM as a form of contraception is most effective when you use multiple methods to identify your fertile days (e.g. cycle tracking, checking temperature and analysing cervical mucus). For the first four weeks after delivery, these fertility signs aren't detectable. Guidance from the UK's FSRH states that if you *are not* breastfeeding, fertility awareness can be used from four weeks after delivery and once you've had three regular menstrual cycles, but that before then, and while breastfeeding (if you don't meet the LAM criteria), you'll need to consider another option.[9]

Just like LAM, you have to be really on the ball to use this method and be extremely diligent about accurately logging your symptoms. For instance, logging your waking basal body temperature (BBT) at the same time every day can be tricky when your sleep routine is often disrupted. Even people who ordinarily had menstrual cycles like clockwork pre-pregnancy can have rogue months, which throw timings out the window. This means you may ovulate earlier or later than expected, making you potentially fertile when you may not think you are. Factors that can play havoc with ovulation include feeling stressed, run-down or sleep-deprived (hello parenthood).

## Sterilisation

If you are having a planned C-section, sterilisation can be booked in so that it happens during your C-section surgery – multitasking at its finest. It would all need to be discussed with your obstetrician in advance, with consent given at least two weeks before your C-section. See page 99 for more on female sterilisation.

## The coil

In the UK, guidelines state that either the copper (IUD) or the hormonal coil (IUS) can be inserted within the first forty-eight hours after delivery, including straight after the placenta has been delivered, or during a C-section if the delivery was uncomplicated. However, in practice, not all maternity services have the capacity or staff with the training to provide this, so during your antenatal care, ask your midwife or doctor whether this is an option.

Having a coil fitted in the postpartum period and while breastfeeding has been associated with an increased risk of damage to the uterus known as perforation. However, coils fitted immediately after an uncomplicated birth, at the time of a C-section or within forty-eight hours of a vaginal birth have been shown to be safe. If you miss this forty-eight-hour window or develop an infection after delivery, the insertion should be delayed until four weeks after (and after any infection has been treated). If you're breastfeeding, or within thirty-six weeks after delivery, you're more likely to have a perforation with a coil, although the risk is still small.[10] Some women are happy with this risk, others prefer to wait and use a different method in the meantime.

Advantages of an early insertion after a vaginal delivery

include less pain on insertion; however, you have to weigh this up against the disadvantage that the coil has a higher risk of falling out (expulsion).[11] Insertion of a coil during a C-section has a lower risk of expulsion, and you'll be numb, so no pain is a bonus.[12] Due to the increased risk of issues with the coil falling out, and sometimes long threads or threads that are difficult to find, if you've had the coil inserted within forty-eight hours of delivery you should have a routine check-up four to six weeks later.[13]

### Emergency contraception

You may want to consider emergency contraception if you have unprotected sex more than twenty-one days after giving birth. Your options are the emergency contraceptive pill or the copper coil. In Chapter 8, we looked at the effects of using emergency contraception while breastfeeding. While a small amount of hormones from the levonorgestrel emergency contraceptive pill may pass into breast milk, it is not harmful to your baby. This means that you can continue to breastfeed after you've taken it.

ellaOne is a different type of emergency contraceptive pill containing ulipristal acetate. Its safety during breastfeeding has only recently been studied. Previously, it was advised to avoid breastfeeding for a week after using ellaOne by expressing and discarding milk for seven days after taking it. However, new research has shown that ellaOne is now considered safe while breastfeeding.[14] For more on this, go back to page 232.

The copper coil is the most effective form of emergency contraception. It is safe to have inserted if you are breastfeeding, taking into account the small increased risk of perforation and depending on general suitability. It can also be continued as a longer-term contraceptive option. If you need emergency contraception between twenty-one and twenty-eight days postpartum there is an increased risk of perforation with the copper coil so this will need to be considered on an individual basis with your healthcare professional.[15]

## Is it postpartum depression or your contraception?

Feeling sad, tearful, anxious and irritable? Or have low energy, a change in appetite and negative thoughts? For some we're describing being on the pill, for others, this feels more akin to postpartum depression. As we looked at in Chapter 5, contraception and mood side effects are consistently reported on The Lowdown, despite much conflicting research around whether contraception could be the root cause. As there are so many other factors that can have a negative impact on a person's mood, it's hard to reach one conclusion. Throw having a baby into the mix, and your hormones have just stepped into overdrive. Around one in seven women experience postpartum depression,[16] a form of depression that impacts the ability to bond with your newborn and can have a huge impact on being able to function day-to-day. Unlike the 'baby blues', postpartum depression persists for longer than two weeks, with some research suggesting it could last for years for some.[17] Every mother should be screened for mood or anxiety symptoms at the postnatal check and pretty much every time you see a midwife or health visitor, but sometimes women can put on a brave face, or the more subtle symptoms may go unnoticed.

Spotting the signs of postpartum depression isn't always easy when you're in the thick of it. Symptoms can come on gradually, and it's often not until a loved one mentions it that you realise you may have it at all. The main symptoms include:[18]

- Feeling sad, low mood and often being tearful.
- Feeling agitated or irritable towards others.
- No longer enjoying things you used to, and losing interest in most things.
- Constant fatigue and tiredness.
- Trouble sleeping at night – even when your baby is sleeping.
- Brain fog, having trouble making decisions.
- An increase or decrease in appetite.
- Feeling like you're not a good enough parent, feeling unable to look after your baby or that your baby doesn't love you.
- Feeling guilt, hopelessness and blaming yourself for everything.
- Feeling anxious that something bad may happen to your baby.
- Problems bonding with your baby, no sense of enjoyment in being with them.

Postpartum depression can impact either parent, and it's thought that you're more likely to experience it if you have a previous history of depression or psychiatric illness, felt depressed during pregnancy or experienced pregnancy complications, don't have a strong support network of family and friends, are from a low socio-economic background or experience a stressful life event after birth.[19] It's important to remember that there is no shame in seeking help for postpartum depression, you are a great parent and your baby still adores you. Please see where you can access support in the Resources section.

**Progestogen-only/mini pill**
Used for 1–3 months 32 years old

★☆☆☆☆

**Cerazette pill**

I took this after my second child in 2019. And it wasn't until my husband thought I had postpartum depression that I realised that this really doesn't agree with me. I struggled with my mental health, I felt sad and overwhelmed all the time. I didn't have my normal drive to get things done or the patience to deal with the children.

Shared on **thelowdown.com**

## Does hormonal contraception increase your risk of having postpartum depression?

If you've previously used contraception and felt it negatively impacted your mood, or you're trying it for the first time after giving birth, you might be worried about potential side effects while you're entering a new (and incredibly busy) phase of your life. One study investigated the link between mood side effects of hormonal contraception and postnatal depression in almost 200,000 first-time mums.[20] It found that if women had suffered from depression related to hormonal contraception in the past, they were more likely to have postpartum depression compared to women who had depression without synthetic hormones being a factor. This may tell us that some women are more sensitive to changes in hormone levels and this impacts their mood.

When it comes to specific contraceptive methods, the

available research on hormonal contraception and postpartum depression shows conflicting evidence. At this stage, are we surprised? A 2019 systematic review[21] highlighted one study which compared combined hormonal contraception, progestogen-only pills, the implant and the hormonal coil alongside people who didn't use hormonal contraception. It found a 35–44 per cent decreased risk of postpartum depression with the progestogen-only pill and hormonal coil, a small increased risk of postpartum antidepressant use among women who used the implant and the vaginal ring, and a decreased risk of antidepressant use with the progestogen-only pill. Another review of research suggested that progestogen-only methods of contraception *are not* associated with higher instances of postpartum depression,[22] and another paper states there *might* be a link between all hormonal contraceptives and postpartum depression.[23] Confusing eh?

Some research even looks at the timing of postpartum contraceptives and mood symptoms. One study found women in South Africa who used the Noristerat injection (which isn't commonly prescribed in the UK any more) immediately after birth were two to three times more likely to experience depression at six weeks, but not at three months postpartum, when rates of depression were equal to women using no contraception at all.[24] Overall, there's been no consistent link found between using hormonal contraceptives and the risk of experiencing postpartum depression – so we just don't know the answer. But if you notice that you're feeling irritable, feel unable to bond with your baby, can't stop crying or have suicidal thoughts or hallucinations, speak to your GP.

### Managing hormonal contraceptive side effects while navigating postpartum life

As we explored in Chapter 5, some of the most common hormonal contraceptive side effects include low sex drive and changes to weight, mood, skin and bleeding patterns. All, rather unhelpfully, things you'll probably juggle in postpartum life anyway. But if you've got additional side effects, it can really add to the relentlessness of the fourth trimester (recent catchphrase in mum culture to describe the first three months postpartum). As we learnt earlier, spacing between pregnancies is important for you and your future baby's health, so if you decide to stop a method, research an alternative or invest in good condoms. It may also be tempting to just put up with side effects, and concentrate your all on this tiny human you are keeping alive. But you do really need to prioritise yourself and fill your cup first, because if you are happy and thriving, your baby will be too. So get on the phone and call the GP if your side effects are making motherhood tougher.

**Hormonal coil (IUS)**
Used for 18 months to 3 years · 32 years old

★★★★★

**Mirena coil**

I used this contraception for the first time after having my second child, so it is hard to say what were side effects of the contraception and what were postpartum side effects. Overall, it was less hard on my system than the pill and preferable to the copper IUD.

Shared on **thelowdown.com**

# 11

# Perimenopause and menopause

So, you've survived your reproductive years. You've made a dent in countless packets of painkillers to manage your periods, tried out multiple contraceptives to find one that works best for you – or perhaps you've been through pregnancy or childbirth. But it's not over *just* yet. There are a few more years of hormonal fluctuations to get through (perimenopause) before your periods stop (menopause).

If you're reading this in your teens, twenties or thirties, or even your forties, and think, 'This doesn't apply to me', stick with us. The earlier we all start to learn about and understand perimenopause, the better prepared we'll be when it happens to us, or to someone we love. Time and time again women tell us that they wish they'd had better sex education aged sixteen, to prepare them for the experiences they are facing at twenty-six. Think of this chapter as a school sex education lesson for adults; it will really help you prepare for what's coming up. Lack of education earlier in life, accessible information and general social awareness has caused perimenopausal women to go through this period of their life with minimal support, perpetuating another generation who feel less able to advocate for themselves because they have no idea what the hell is happening to them. Let's change that.

Perimenopause can be a time of huge upheaval for those going through it, with a wide range of physical and emotional symptoms to navigate. We have a rising number of women over forty-five in the UK, therefore the conversation surrounding perimenopause needs to be high on the public health agenda.

Historically, as with so many areas of women's health, menopause has been a taboo subject. Which is why, in 2024, we expanded our contraception review platform into menopause, so women can share their experiences, symptoms and satisfaction rating across every regimen of hormone replacement therapy (HRT) and non-hormonal treatments that are currently used to treat perimenopausal and menopausal symptoms in the UK. We've heard countless stories of women who've had to battle through horrendous symptoms and diminished quality of life only to be dismissed or misdiagnosed. Limited research on this stage of life was available, which meant many healthcare professionals did not have the know-how needed to help women through it. The great news is that mindsets, medical understanding and treatments are changing rapidly, and for the better.

And we have an opportunity to speak out too, to continue to demand better. Rather than 'women of a certain age' becoming invisible, we need to insist on more research and greater support. We need change from employers supporting perimenopausal and postmenopausal staff to healthcare professionals receiving more training on treatments for this stage of life. Our mothers, grandmothers and generations before them were badly let down to suffer in silence. Let's make sure we have a better perimenopause than they did!

This chapter looks at the pathway from our thirties and

early forties to perimenopause, including how to spot perimenopause starting along with what the treatment options are, as lots of women we've spoken to are surprised that symptoms can start as early as this. We'll be exploring why contraception during this time can be just as important as previous years, what you can expect going from perimenopausal to postmenopausal, and how that can impact contraception needs.

## What is perimenopause?

Perimenopause is a phase of life that every woman and person assigned female at birth goes through. It's a natural transition that results from fluctuating hormones in our body, and usually happens over several years. The term 'menopause' actually only marks one date in the calendar – one whole year since a person, over forty-five, has had their last period. The time leading up to this red-letter day is known as 'perimenopause'. After your periods stop, you're 'postmenopausal'.

Over the course of your perimenopausal years, oestrogen levels in your body fluctuate wildly before declining, often resulting in physical and emotional changes. The start of perimenopause is hard to define but is usually when you start experiencing symptoms from these changes. It can make you feel like you're in a never-ending PMS nightmare, along with symptoms as serious as anxiety and depression. On page 305, we'll look at the many reported symptoms of perimenopause, which can differ greatly between individuals. Some may not have any symptoms at all but the majority of us do, ranging from mild to severe. Four out of five postmenopausal women experience hot flushes, a quarter have very few or no symptoms and around a quarter report a severe impact on quality of life, with the rest of us somewhere in the middle.[1] For some, symptoms come and go, while others find they don't get much let-up. They can also become more or less intense until menopause is reached and beyond.

It doesn't sound great, does it? Rest assured, there is positive news as there are lots of treatment options that can greatly reduce these side effects. Later in this chapter we'll be taking a close look at hormone replacement therapy (HRT) as well as hormonal contraception, and how these can work wonders to ease many of the symptoms of perimenopause.

## The hormones of perimenopause

Ask Dr Google what's going on during perimenopause and you'll likely read vague descriptions about oestrogen levels being in decline during this time. Even one of the go-to treatments for perimenopausal symptoms is called hormone *replacement* therapy. This terminology suggests our hormones need topping up. But actually, it's not so simple. Hormones pulse through our bodies up and down, rather than ever being in a level state. During perimenopause, progesterone levels initially begin to fall, which can affect your periods and sleep pattern. As the number of eggs in the ovaries reduces, oestrogen levels fluctuate with huge peaks and deep troughs, which causes problems such as hot flushes, headaches and irritability. Your overall levels of oestrogen and progesterone (along with testosterone) gradually decrease until they reach a baseline level at menopause. Then you shrivel up into a fossil and vaporise . . . of course not. But some societal attitudes towards menopausal women would have you believe otherwise.

## Hormonal fluctuations by age

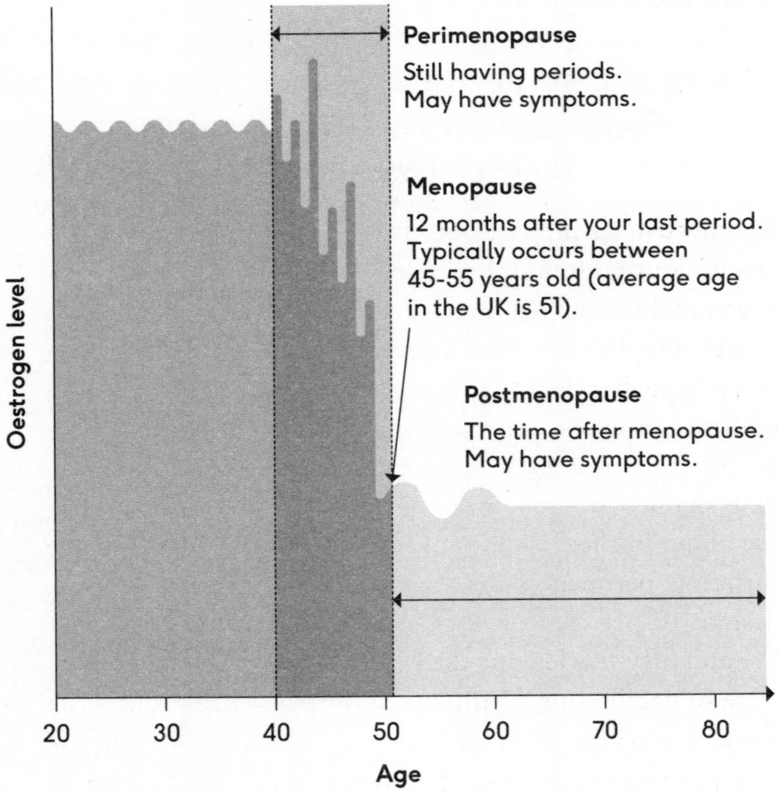


## When is perimenopause and how long will it last?

There are no fixed timings with perimenopause – it can start at different ages and can last varying lengths of time, from just a few months to more than thirteen years for some.[2] Usually, though, it begins around your mid-forties and lasts an average of four to eight years before menopause,[3] for which the average age in the UK is fifty-one.[4] During this time, symptoms may come and go, with stages where things feel worse and other times where your symptoms improve or disappear. The unpredictable nature of perimenopause means it's tricky to navigate; fortunately, though, there are lifestyle changes and treatments available that can help.

**When do I need to start thinking about perimenopause?**

So, how can we prepare ourselves? A study by the *Women's Health* journal found that 90 per cent of women had never been taught about the menopause at school, and more than 60 per cent didn't feel informed about it at all.[5] How, when there is such a lack of information about our changing bodies, can we be expected to prepare for this transition? So often it's this lack of proper education and guidance that shames women into silence, or into thinking they are alone in their symptoms. Only around half of people suffering perimenopausal symptoms speak to their GP, despite 10 per cent of women between the ages of forty-five and fifty-five leaving their jobs because their symptoms were so debilitating.[6] Millions of other women around the world are trying to muddle through as best they can, as they have no other option but to keep working. Talking to others around you, especially those who have been through perimenopause, means you'll be able to make informed choices when the time comes.

## Symptoms

Ever wondered how long a piece of string is? The list of perimenopausal symptoms is lengthy and varies a lot between individuals (in terms of both the symptoms and how they are experienced). In medical literature, you'll sometimes see it written that there are thirty-four symptoms of the menopause and perimenopause, but there are more. In a survey by the British Menopause Society, the average number of symptoms a person has is seven.[7] Here are some of these common ones (but this list is sadly not exhaustive!):

- Changes to your period – this could be cycle length with longer or shorter times between periods, and heavier or lighter flow lasting for more or fewer days.
- Hot flushes – affecting 80 per cent of perimenopausal women.[8]
- Changes to your sleep pattern.
- Breast pain.
- Cyclical headaches.
- Palpitations.
- Anxiety.
- Mood changes.
- Irritability.
- Fatigue.
- Skin and hair changes.
- Joint and muscle pain.
- Genital or urinary symptoms (e.g. vaginal dryness, painful sex and urine infections).
- Loss of libido.

If these aren't unpleasant enough, the knock-on impact of feeling so rough can be emotionally exhausting.

**Unsure if perimenopausal**
Started less than 1 year ago · 41 years old

I am almost forty-two and experiencing perimenopause – this has not been diagnosed by a GP. It has been more noticeable in the past six months. The most severe symptom is the irregularity and heaviness of my periods, along with bloating. My skin and hair feel worse – recurrent breakouts along with hair thinning. I am trying to exercise regularly and I find this improves my mood.

Shared on **thelowdown.com**

### How to tell if 'side effects' from contraception are actually the first signs of perimenopause

It's not always easy to tell if how you're feeling is linked to perimenopause or due to the everyday stresses of life. Sometimes women start to notice symptoms that feel just a bit 'off', and period changes are often one of the most obvious signs that people report first.

During perimenopause, you'll still have periods but they often change during this time, becoming heavier or lighter, longer or shorter and generally more irregular. This is down to an initial drop in progesterone levels. At the same time, oestrogen levels fluctuate up and down while the ovaries continue to try to release the limited number of remaining eggs.

While changes to your periods may be a sign you're perimenopausal, you can also be perimenopausal with regular periods. Confused? That's understandable. Generally, as perimenopause is reaching an end, the length of time between your periods gets longer. It doesn't always follow a neat trajectory, though; you might not have a period for months, only for them to start up again. By and large, longer gaps between bleeds usually suggest you're heading towards them stopping altogether.

### Do contraceptive side effects change as you get older anyway?

Guess what – there's pretty much no research into this, but it's a story we hear all the time at The Lowdown. Women who have been happy on their contraceptive for years start to notice new side effects or symptoms. We see this as women get older and move into perimenopause, and also hear that side effects can completely change after pregnancy.

---

**Q:** I've struggled with my cycle since I was a teenager. Terrible PMS each month along with painful periods. Does this mean perimenopause symptoms will be severe for me?

**A:** There's limited research into this at the moment. But we do believe that the hormonal changes in perimenopause may cause worse symptoms in women who already have hormonally sensitive conditions, such as PMS and PMDD.[9] It's important to be aware of this so you can discuss it with your healthcare professional early on if you're concerned.

---

## Diagnosing perimenopause

If you're over the age of forty-five, perimenopause should be diagnosed clinically, meaning it will be based on symptoms rather than a test. So, it's really useful to track your symptoms, keeping a record that you can show to your healthcare professional. This can help your doctor assess whether you're experiencing early signs of perimenopause or if there is something else at play. Being armed with a list can also help kickstart the conversation with your healthcare professional more easily; see our symptom checker in Resources.

A blood test for follicle stimulating hormone (FSH) levels, which are raised in postmenopausal women, is unreliable during perimenopause because your hormones fluctuate constantly. Because a blood test would only show the hormonal level on that particular day and not the overall picture, it's often unhelpful for those who have typical perimenopausal symptoms over the age of forty-five.

The exceptions to this are if you are under the age of forty-five with perimenopausal symptoms, or if you are over fifty and on progestogen-only contraception which stops your periods, and want to know if you can stop taking it.[10] In these cases, FSH testing may help your doctor or nurse decide if you are perimenopausal and also when to stop using contraception. (See Chapter 7 on stopping and switching.) Whatever your age, if you suspect you are in perimenopause, and would like information and support, speak to a healthcare professional.

### Premature ovarian insufficiency and early menopause

If you're under forty and have perimenopausal symptoms or absent/irregular periods for four months or longer (and not as a result of hormonal contraception), you should be investigated for primary ovarian insufficiency (POI). This is sometimes called premature ovarian failure or premature menopause. Two blood tests will be carried out four to six weeks apart to assess FSH, which rises during perimenopause and stays raised post menopause. Less than 1 per cent of women will become menopausal before the age of forty, and likely less than 0.1

per cent under the age of thirty.[11] However, if left untreated, premature ovarian insufficiency and early menopause (menopause between the ages of forty and forty-five) can impact your long-term health, so receiving an accurate and timely diagnosis is key to getting the right support.

In most cases POI is idiopathic, meaning there is no known cause. Genes and family history may play a part in early menopause, so you could have a chat with family members about their experience of perimenopause. You might find your symptoms and timings to be similar to theirs, but there's no way to predict exactly when it'll begin for you. There are also certain medical conditions and treatments that can cause perimenopause and menopause to start early, such as autoimmune conditions, genetic conditions such as Turner syndrome, or treatments including surgery to remove the ovaries, chemotherapy or pelvic radiotherapy.

---

**Q:** Can you still get pregnant if you have POI? Do I still need contraception?

We asked Dr Nikki Ramskill, The Lowdown clinical lead and founder of The Female Doctor Clinic. Nikki was diagnosed with POI aged thirty-seven . . .

**A:** 'The short answer is yes you can. There is around a 5–10 per cent chance of natural conception because POI is different to menopause.[12] The ovaries intermittently function, rather than a complete shut-down, so some months ovulation could occur. All women with POI are advised to use contraception if they don't wish to get pregnant. There are many safe options that can be used up to the age of fifty-five, when all women (even those without POI) can stop using it.'

---

**I'm post menopausal**
Started 10+ years ago    33 years old

I started my menstrual cycle at the age of 11, and up until I was 27 years of age it had always been regular. I started noticing that I was becoming irregular, missing months here and there. I went to my GP who carried out a series of blood tests. One of which was the FSH (Follicle Stimulating Hormone) blood test. The result[s] were high and the doctor stated she would repeat them in two weeks which she did. This time the results weren't high and it had come down. She sent me away and told me that there wasn't anything to worry about and to keep an eye on my iron levels. During this time I'm suffering with very bad anxiety but I couldn't pin point it. I thought it may have been triggered from a bad flight I had taken. I'm now 33, and my [menstrual]cycle has become irregular again. The FSH blood test was repeated and showing a high reading. This time I had been referred to a specialist hospital [for] a scan and more blood tests. The consultant came into the room with a folder in his hand, as he walked to his chair he looked at me over his glasses and said 'You're in the menopause'.

Shared on **thelowdown.com**

## Could your contraception be masking symptoms of perimenopause?

Contraception doesn't kickstart menopause or have any effect on its timeline, but what if the contraceptive you are using is masking the symptoms of your last period? People who use progestogen-only contraceptives may experience amenorrhoea (stopped periods), and as we've discussed in Chapter 2, bleeds on combined contraception aren't true periods. So in that case how would you know if you're going through perimenopause?

Measuring FSH levels is one option for people using progestogen-only methods over the age of fifty. In this case, if the FSH levels are raised, women can stop contraception one year later without needing to retest.[13]

Those using combined hormonal contraception (pills, patch or vaginal ring) or hormone replacement therapy (HRT) have suppressed levels of certain hormones (oestrogen and FSH); therefore, testing is not recommended as it does not give any accurate information. You'll be advised to stop combined hormonal contraception and the contraceptive injection by the age of fifty anyway, and to switch to the hormonal coil, implant, progestogen-only pill or a non-hormonal option.[14]

## Hormone replacement therapy

While this book is about contraception, we couldn't have a chapter on perimenopause and menopause without a nod to hormone replacement therapy (HRT). HRT is a natural progression from contraception for many women, which is why we expanded The Lowdown to include HRT reviews on our website. At least 15 per cent of women aged forty-five to sixty-four in England use HRT[15] as a way to manage their menopausal symptoms, and this figure is rising. This may be an important part of your future, so it's worth learning about early.

Standard HRT contains two hormones: oestrogen and progesterone. It's the oestrogen which generally helps the symptoms of perimenopause. However, if you have a uterus, oestrogen can cause the uterus lining to overgrow, which can increase your risk of cancer of the uterus. To protect against this, progesterone is used alongside the oestrogen to keep the uterus lining thin. This is called 'endometrial protection'. It's really important that you use both the oestrogen and progesterone together if you have a uterus. The progesterone part is taken continuously every day (to avoid a monthly bleed) or cyclically for ten to fourteen days a month (to cause a monthly bleed). Your healthcare professional will discuss which is the right option for you. HRT that treats your whole body (also called systemic HRT) is available on prescription and comes in different forms, whereas vaginal oestrogen is a type of localised HRT and can be prescribed or bought in pharmacies.

Many people find HRT is incredible at alleviating the symptoms of perimenopause, from problematic periods and hot flushes to low mood and anxiety (to name a few). Some women find it literally life changing. There are also long-term benefits associated with taking it, like protecting bone, heart and blood vessel health.

**HRT review**

Used for more than 12 months   53 years old

★★★★★

I changed doctors to get the HRT I wanted. Luckily, we moved areas but this shows how different my experience could be according to postcode. HRT has changed my life irrevocably and I really don't feel I could live without it, nor do I want to. I really felt like my life was over at fifty and now I have started a new business, am supporting my children (one of whom is autistic) and enjoying a healthy social life, as well as a healthy marriage. I truly believe I couldn't manage any of this without HRT.

Shared on **thelowdown.com**

However, other people have less positive experiences using HRT, where it can actually cause side effects, in addition to perimenopausal symptoms, that make them feel even worse. In this aspect, it's so similar to hormonal contraception in that there are many different doses and regimens of HRT, and sometimes it's a trial-and-error process to find your perfect fit. And just like some hormonal contraception, HRT is not suitable for everyone. This is due to some small risks associated with it, mainly for women with a history of breast cancer.

**I'm perimenopausal**

Started 1–3 years ago    44 years old

My symptoms started eighteen months ago and I've been through various scans and tests for my period issues (heavy, long, painful) where nothing untoward is identified but in the meantime I'm still experiencing all the symptoms. I finally asked the GP for HRT, but they wouldn't prescribe it due to mum's family history of breast cancer twice, so, yet again, had to wait for another referral back to community gynae. I had my appointment yesterday and agreement for HRT and having the Mirena coil, which I've got to wait another six to eight weeks for, but in the meantime I can be prescribed vaginal estrogen for dryness and pain and bleeding during sex, so I can start that this week. I work for the NHS so am pretty aware of and have read up on perimenopause and referrals etc., but I do think I could have been started on HRT much sooner, when I first reported my symptoms eighteen months ago. That, I think, would have been helping me by now. I'm looking forward to this next phase in my life as I just want to get my symptoms under control.

Shared on **thelowdown.com**

So, how can you weigh up whether HRT is right for you? While your doctor will assess your medical suitability before prescribing it, you will also need to assess the pros and cons (just like using hormonal contraceptives or any other medication). If you decide it's not the approach for you, there are other options out there.

One final thing to remember about HRT is that it's not a contraceptive. In fact, one study found that perimenopausal women who weren't ovulating before starting HRT then went on to ovulate, thus increasing their chance of pregnancy.[16] So don't forget about contraception just yet.

## Contraception and perimenopause

At The Lowdown, we talk a lot about the importance of being clued up on contraception – and this goes for people in their forties and fifties, too. Contraception can continue to have many uses during the perimenopausal years that aren't just for preventing pregnancy. However, as we age we are at increasing risk of some health conditions. This means that choosing appropriate contraception requires an understanding of the health benefits and risks of each method, and the non-contraceptive advantages and disadvantages for this age group. So, let's take a closer look at the scenarios when hormonal contraception is used by women in their forties and fifties.

### Contraception for preventing pregnancy

Yes, society, perimenopausal women do have sex! If you are perimenopausal, even if your periods are all over the place, you can still get pregnant. An unplanned pregnancy at an older age can be a complete shock, but it's possible.

While men continue to produce sperm into old age, we know

that women's fertility declines with age. With press headlines telling us our fertility 'falls off a cliff' after our mid-thirties and expectant mothers over thirty-five still sometimes labelled 'geriatric', it's no wonder many perimenopausal women falsely assume they can no longer get pregnant. While pregnancy may be less likely, at the age of forty, 44 per cent of couples having unprotected sex will get pregnant within a year.[17] However, pregnancies that do occur after forty years old have an increased risk of adverse outcomes for both mother and child, including miscarriage, gestational diabetes and pre-eclampsia.[18]

It may be tempting to stop using contraception in your forties and fifties, with the assumption that your fertility has reduced, but if you want to avoid pregnancy, you are advised to continue using contraception until you are postmenopausal (see page 322). So let's look at what the most suitable options are, taking into account the associated health risks.

*Hormonal contraception*

The combined pill, patch and ring can be used up to the age of fifty, after which there is a concern regarding the risks associated with it (see Chapter 6) and so switching to a safer alternative is advised.

The contraceptive injection (Depo Provera and Sayana Press) is also associated with a small decrease in bone mineral density which can increase the risk of osteoporosis (i.e. thinning of the bones). The risk of getting osteoporosis increases as you get older anyway, therefore, if you are over forty and using the injection you should be reviewed regularly to assess the benefits and risks. Those over fifty should consider alternative methods of contraception.[19]

If you're using one of the 52 mg levonorgestrel hormonal coils (Mirena, Levosert and Benilexa) for contraception and it was inserted when you were forty-five or older you can keep this in until the age of fifty-five to protect against pregnancy. However, this still needs to be changed every five years if you're using it as part of HRT.[20] The progestogen-only pill, implant and lower dose coils (Kyleena and Jaydess) are safe to use throughout perimenopause and up until the age of fifty-five with very few risks. They may even help bleeding symptoms from perimenopause too.

If you're using HRT, you can't have combined contraception alongside, but all forms of progestogen-only contraception are safe to use at the same time as HRT.

*Other options*

If you're someone who prefers non-hormonal methods of contraception, you might be wondering if they're still an option for this stage of life. Let's see:

- **Barrier methods** Condoms, caps and diaphragms can continue to be used effectively and condoms will help protect against sexually transmitted diseases (STIs).
- **Fertility awareness methods (FAM, i.e. natural family planning)** This isn't recommended during perimenopause because signs like cycle length, waking temperature and cervical fluid become less reliable markers during perimenopause. This can make it a higher risk method than before perimenopause if you were able to predictably track your cycle. If you're using HRT, you can't rely on FAM because it can throw your fertility signs into disarray.
- **Copper coil** Copper coils that have a copper content of 300 mm$^2$ can be left in until menopause when inserted aged forty or over.[21] In reality, this is every brand of copper coil apart from the GyneFix 200 (which is rarely used in the UK). Copper coils are really popular, but be wary that their main potential side effect of heavy, prolonged periods may worsen during perimenopause.

- **Sterilisation** Female sterilisation is a surgical procedure whereby the fallopian tubes are sealed or blocked, preventing pregnancy by stopping eggs and sperm from meeting. It can still be an option if you're perimenopausal, bearing in mind your medical suitability and the small risks (see page 200). Sterilisation won't have any impact on the hormones of the menopause and it can be carried out while using hormonal contraceptives or HRT.

## Contraception to manage perimenopausal symptoms

Just as contraception can be brilliant at alleviating period side effects, it can be as effective with perimenopausal symptoms. As we know, the erratic hormonal changes during perimenopause can cause a long list of unwelcome physical and emotional changes, and combined hormonal contraception (the pill, patch and ring), especially when taken continuously, can help to flatten those peaks and troughs. The hormonal coil and sometimes other progestogen-based methods (the progestogen-only pill, injection and implant) can reduce menstrual bleeding and pain associated with periods in the perimenopause.

We asked our friends Dr Olivia Hum and Dr Zoe Schaedel, GPs and menopause specialists from Myla Health, to answer some of our most frequently asked questions relating to perimenopause. You'll find their answers in each of the Q & A's in the rest of this chapter:

---

**Q:** Which brands of combined contraception are the best to use during perimenopause?

**A:** 'There is no evidence to say one brand is any "better" than another when it comes to managing perimenopause symptoms. Some women prefer to use a brand which contains body-identical oestrogen (like Zoely or Qlaira) rather than the synthetic ethinylestradiol in most combined pills.'

---

Using a combined contraceptive can also help protect you from osteoporosis as it helps to supplement the oestrogen levels in your body. The loss of bone mineral density is a concern in perimenopausal women as it can increase the risk of fractures and bone pain. But it's important to know that HRT is better than the combined pill at preventing bone density loss,[22] and combined contraceptives should only be used up until the age of fifty (provided your medical history and risk factors allow).

---

**Q:** Will the progestogen-only pill help my perimenopause symptoms?

**A:** 'It depends what the symptoms are. Some of the symptoms of perimenopause are caused by the instability of hormones at that time. This is particularly an issue for women with hormonal migraines. Taking the progestogen-only pill can stabilise hormones and stop the ups and downs. It can also, in many women, reduce or stop heavy or painful periods. If your symptoms are due to lack of oestrogen then the progestogen-only pill will not help, and for some women it can have side effects, like irregular bleeding or mood changes.'

---

## Contraception as part of HRT

If you're considering HRT and still need contraception, there are some handy contraceptive options that can be used as part of your HRT regimen. Hormonal coils that contain 52 mg of the progestogen levonorgestrel (Mirena, Levosert and Benilexa) can be used to provide endometrial protection alongside oestrogen as part of HRT. We mentioned earlier that extended use of the hormonal coil until age fifty-five is supported if inserted at forty-five years or older for contraceptive purposes; remember, though, that if it is being used as part of your HRT, it must be changed every five years. This makes sure the progestogen dose remains high enough to protect the uterus lining against the effects of oestrogen in HRT, and there has been no research yet to support that there is still enough progestogen after five years to do this. The hormonal coils are also great options for perimenopausal bleeding symptoms, as 73 per cent of The Lowdown users who reviewed the hormonal coil reported it stopped or lightened their periods,[23] and our HRT reviewers also find it a great option.

**HRT review**
Used for more than 12 months · 53 years old

★★★★☆

I found that utrogestan and oestrogel together weren't stopping the incredibly heavy (on occasion debilitatingly so), long periods and bleeding. After trying different doses, in the end the Mirena coil was fitted and stopped the bleeding, improved other symptoms and made me wish someone had suggested it earlier.

Shared on **thelowdown.com**

For some women, menopause specialists may consider using progestogen-only pills, possibly at different doses, for endometrial protection, but this is off licence.

---

**Q:** What are the risks of taking HRT in perimenopause?

**A:** 'Very little research has been done on perimenopause, and there is still some controversy about when perimenopause starts and how it is defined. All the evidence we have about HRT and its risks and benefits comes from research in postmenopausal women. There is some evidence that taking contraception containing a progestogen very slightly increases the risk of breast cancer (see Chapter 6, page 183) but this is about all we have! We know that taking any oral oestrogen (including some types of HRT or the combined pill) can increase the risks of having a blood clot. This is a small increased risk at any age, but the risks do increase with age, so it may be more suitable for some women to use HRT through the skin (transdermal). Irregular bleeding is a common side effect – and not all women feel great taking HRT in perimenopause – some just feel very hormonal and find that it makes the hormonal instability worse.'

---

## How to tell if perimenopause is ending?

It isn't always obvious when you're coming to the end of perimenopause. This is because symptoms can come and go, increasing and decreasing in severity. So, rather than assessing it on symptoms, the medical definition of perimenopause ending is when you haven't had a period for twelve months. When the gaps between your periods get longer, it usually suggests perimenopause is coming to an end. You can be thrown some curveballs, though – like no periods for eleven months, only to have one again, meaning your twelve-month countdown to menopause starts all over again.

## Menopause

So, 365 days have passed since your last period. For some people, this is a mega milestone, a day that can carry a huge range of emotions from celebration, relief and pride. But it's also totally normal to feel grief, sadness or overwhelm as you move from one key phase of life to the next.

From the day after 'menopause', you're clinically described as postmenopausal. After menopause, your baseline hormones are lower than during your reproductive years. Menopause doesn't mark the end of your symptoms, and you may continue to experience them. For this reason, it's a good idea to look after yourself in all the usual ways – a nutritious balanced diet, trying to keep fit, etc. Fortunately, if you are using treatments such as HRT, you can continue to take them with an annual medical review to ensure it's still a suitable option for you.

### Saying goodbye to contraception altogether

The advice is to continue using contraception until you're menopausal. In reality, this means you can safely stop contraception:

- Two years after your last period if you are aged forty to fifty.
- One year after your last period if you are aged over fifty.
- If you are over the age of fifty-five when the natural loss of fertility can be assumed (pregnancy over the age

of fifty-five is extremely rare even if women are still having periods).

Remember, though, to prevent catching or spreading a sexually transmitted infection (STI), condoms should still be used if needed. STIs are on the up in all ages, including middle and older age![24] So it's important to have STI screening if you change sexual partner.

# 12

# The future of contraception

Writing this book over the course of 2024, our publisher expressed concern that this chapter would date quickly. How optimistic, we thought! Unfortunately, at The Lowdown we feel that the problem is it *won't*. There has been very little innovation and investment in the development of new contraceptive methods globally, and while this chapter will share some of the incredible advancements that researchers are working on, we need many more options (for both men and women) *and* quicker progress to get them tested and safely into the market.

The advent of the pill in the 1960s was revolutionary, but as we saw in Chapter 3, there have been surprisingly few contraceptive developments since then. Hormonal methods like the contraceptive pill, patch, ring, injection and implant all work in basically the same way. When developing the pill, scientists put their focus on preventing pregnancy by suppressing the menstrual cycle, without fully understanding its complexity.[1] In fact, there is still so much to learn about female reproductive health, we've barely scratched the surface of the potential for developing other approaches to preventing pregnancy.

So, why have there been so many breakthroughs in other areas of health but not contraceptives? There seems to be a view held by large pharmaceutical companies that investing in new and improved contraceptives isn't worth it – that uptake would be low and potential revenue limited. We believe otherwise and we know that public demand has the power to rally a mindset change. So, in this chapter we look at how we can do our bit to help progress reproductive well-being by getting involved in research.

What does such a lack of innovation and investment mean? Well, the impact of the contraception deficit is far reaching. Lots of people aren't happy with their method.[2] And when we lack suitable options, we take more risks. Over half of the pregnancies that occur worldwide are unintended, which has a significant knock-on impact on abortion rates.[3] Globally, 45 per cent of abortions are unsafe[4] – it's estimated that around 39,000 women die from unsafe abortions every year, with millions hospitalised due to complications.[5] In 2022, abortions in England and Wales reached record levels,[6] and this is a trend also playing out in many other parts of the world. There's an alarming number of adults in the UK having unprotected sex, often because of a misconception around contraceptives or lack of education about them, coupled with issues around accessing contraception, general lack of information and in some parts of society stigma associated with using it. We need greater focus on empowering people through better education around using contraceptives to prevent pregnancy and STIs.

With the global population rising, the climate crisis altering life as we know it and many people's resources squeezed, you could say we've never had a greater need for better contraceptive options. So, what does our contraceptive future hold and can we hope that the best contraceptives are yet to come? In this chapter we give you some reasons to be positive. We explain what users of contraception want, how drug development works and what is being worked on in both male- and female-targeted contraceptives. So, if you've picked this book up several years after publication, the story may not have dramatically moved forward. But if you're reading this a generation from now, the contraceptive landscape will hopefully be transformed.

## What do we want from new methods?

We already know from The Lowdown's contraception review data that overall satisfaction with the methods reviewed isn't great. The average satisfaction rating is 3.2/5[7] (so what our reviewers class as 'average'), which, if you imagine choosing a restaurant with that rating on Google reviews, isn't hugely tantalising.

Research suggests that what users of contraception actually want is pretty simple: effectiveness, lack of side effects and affordability.[8] The same study showed that 91 per cent of women found that no contraceptive method encompassed these three all-important criteria. We also hear from women who want more options for longer-lasting methods that don't rely on remembering to do something daily like take a pill. For others, control over administration of a method is important, whereby you can stop and start a method without needing regular trips to a doctor or clinic.

We know what we want from our contraception on the home front, but what about contraceptive needs in other parts of the world? While the data above is taken from a largely UK and US audience, anecdotal and research evidence from across the world shows similar themes. In developing countries, lack of access and worry over side effects are key reasons for unmet need, along with a lack of options and, in some parts of the world, cultural barriers.[9] Many women want or need to be discreet about using contraceptives for a variety of reasons, such as their partner, family or community disapproving. This means that certain methods which can be seen on the body (like the patch) are ruled out,[10] so we need to see more methods that cater to discretion.

In a Lowdown poll, we asked our community if they'd like to see more female or male contraceptives developed and the result was overwhelmingly (you've guessed it): male. Let's get into that more in the next section.

## How does the development of a new drug or medical device work?

Have you heard the old joke about the progress of male contraception? Its arrival has been thirty years away . . . for the last thirty years. Contraception (male and female) is an area of health that is underfunded, for sure. But it's important to understand that the development of *any* drug or medical device takes several years, even decades. So, when we look at the hurdles involved in bringing a new contraceptive to market, it's easier to understand why many of the new methods explored in this chapter are still five to ten years away.

### Research and clinical trials

From over-the-counter pain relief, antibiotics and routine vaccines to medical devices like the hormonal or copper coil, what these all have in common is that they successfully passed extensive research, development and clinical trials. Going from initial concept, pre-clinical lab development and clinical trials to us being able to get our hands on a new medication requires a lot of box-ticking. In fact, far more drugs *don't* make it through to be sold and used in the real world than those that do – only about 10–20 per cent reach us, despite years of research.[11] Because of this low 'success' rate, investors behind the development of new drugs or medical products will always be highly selective about those they choose to fund (which may, annoyingly, explain their caution around the development of male contraceptives).

Any developments in medicine need to be rooted in evidence for them to become part of medical practice or treatment. It's the trialling of a drug or device that leads to evidence (or doesn't, as the case may be). Pre-clinical trials are tests and studies performed before a drug or treatment reaches humans. Think petri dishes, microscopes and lab rats. Their aim is to work out if a drug or treatment can potentially work and be useful. The term 'clinical research' just means any research that involves humans. When lab-based pre-clinical research hits a certain stage, it's deemed ready for the clinical stage. Whether it's a trial to test a new drug or medical device, or research into improving existing medical practices, rigorous research is required. Undertaking medical research and trials requires major financial backing, with funding coming either from public bodies (e.g. governments giving grants to research universities) or privately (e.g. pharmaceutical companies or private organisations).

## Clinical trial phases

While every clinical trial is different in terms of its subject and aims, the key steps followed are the same. Clinical trials for new medications involving human subjects are grouped into three or four different phases, with each subsequent phase building on the learnings of the previous one. The timeline to bring a product through these phases can take many years, with trials stopping early if one of the necessary criteria (like safety and whether it works) can't be proven.

Trials give an opportunity for researchers and developers to prove that their product is safe and effective. Those in charge of the trial also need to prove it's needed and that it's filling an essential gap in the market. Furthermore, trials also have to reach the conclusion that there is a strong benefit to the drug that outweighs potential risk.

- **Phase 1** This involves a small number of healthy volunteers and is the first time the medication is given to anyone. Only small dosages are given at this stage, as researchers monitor the drug's effect on the body as well as any side effects that are experienced.
- **Phase 2** The medication is given to a slightly larger number of volunteers, who the drug is designed for (i.e. to treat their illness or to prevent their ability to conceive).
- **Phase 3** A larger group of people (for whom the drug is designed) are involved at this stage, with some people given the new medication (treatment group) and others given either an existing medication or a placebo (control group). Researchers will analyse how the new drugs fare against the placebo or control group.

For a drug to secure the necessary approvals from the medical regulator, they'll need to see conclusive evidence as part of phases 1–3. It's an exhaustive process that usually takes at least a decade and a casual $800 million-plus budget.[12]

- **Phase 4** If a drug successfully completes phases 1–3, and has been permitted to be marketed and given to patients, then in phase 4 it will continue to be monitored to ensure its safety and efficacy in the long term.

## Get involved in research

Women's health is hugely under-researched and in need of so much more investment. A history of excluding women from research means that we are still under-represented in many studies today. Increased understanding into this area will bring more knowledge of how our bodies work, along with medical conditions and how to treat them. So, you might be wondering if there's anything you can do to help contribute to progress – yes, there is! Getting involved in research is one of the most useful ways the general public can bring more attention to neglected areas of health. From participating in huge randomised controlled trials to filling out a hospital survey about your experience of being treated, it all counts!

Clinical studies always need individuals to take part. Every study has its own list of criteria for who is eligible to participate ('inclusion criteria') and who may not be suitable ('exclusion criteria'). They all vary in terms of what they require from a participant and other details, like the time-frame involved. The level of commitment needed really varies too. At one end of the scale is low-effort, one-time participation; at the other end participants are required to be much more involved and sometimes over a longer period of time, like months or even years. Whatever your availability, you should be able to find some way of getting involved. You might be particularly interested in studies into conditions or side effects that you have direct experience with. It may be possible to find a research study or trial exploring this.

In the Resources (page 362), we list ways to find out about research studies or trials looking for participants. The first step is to reach out and express your interest.

## Male contraception developments

With men statistically likely to earn more cash than women, be promoted ahead of women at work and represent women politically, the lack of contraceptive parity becomes even more stark.[13] Given the last radical innovation in male contraception happened in the nineteenth century (hello, vasectomy), I think we're all more than due the next. Let's find out what's been holding things up and how close we are to more male methods.

## Perceptions around male contraception

There are only two options available for men: condoms and vasectomy. The fact that women's contraception is so much more developed than men's really bucks the trend for women's healthcare, which has historically been much less researched than men's. Despite male contraceptives being studied for many decades, there is no hormonal male contraceptive commercially available. And this isn't necessarily down to an unwillingness on the part of men. But how would you feel about it?

In a poll we conducted, we asked over three thousand women whether they thought their partner would take the male pill or gel: 31 per cent said 'Yes', 48 per cent said 'I think so/maybe' and 21 per cent said 'No'.[14] We also asked if women would be comfortable with their male sexual partner(s) taking responsibility for contraception (specifically the male contraceptive gel as the main form of contraception used). There was a range of responses.

*'I wouldn't because I wouldn't trust him to be responsible.'*

*'I trust my partner completely but we have two children. I'm done. We're done. It would scare me not to have control . . . I guess he trusts me so perhaps I should.'*

*'I'd be worried that guys would use this as another way to pressure women not to use condoms ...'*

*'My boyfriend would probably shower, bathe and moisturise with the gel!'*

Picture the scene: it's 2050 and you've been dating a guy for a little while. You've both had STI checks and have been using condoms as your one and only form of contraception. A couple of months in, he tells you he's just started taking the male pill, so you don't need to use any additional contraception when you have sex. How does it feel to put the responsibility for preventing pregnancy solely in his hands? Any concerns that he may be careless about remembering to take his pill?

With male methods firmly on the horizon, it raises a whole new world of possibilities and challenges. What will the implications be for women with men having more reproductive autonomy? Will we see changes like a decrease in women taking hormonal contraception and a reduction in unintended pregnancies and, in turn, abortion rates? Will women trust men who say they're using hormonal contraception or will many want to see proof, like COVID-style vaccination passports?

After a lifetime of many women taking the lead on contraception, there will definitely be some practicalities to work out. What is promising, though, is how willing both men and women seem to be about new male methods. In Britain, one-third of sexually active men would be open to the idea of taking a male pill, which is around the same percentage of women using hormonal contraception.[15] There's an appetite for a change in the status quo, for shared responsibility and for men having more control over their reproductivity.

### Why is it so damn difficult to create male contraceptives?

We know what you're thinking ... given the dozens of options out there for women, surely it can't be *that* hard to find some for men, right? Well, actually, researchers navigating the field of male contraception face challenges. For the last few decades, quite a bit of research has been undertaken in an attempt to plug the massive gap in male contraception. Here's why it's tricky.

Firstly, there are physiological factors. Women are fertile for a few days each month, usually ovulating around thirteen times per year. In contrast, men are potentially fertile 24/7, 365 days a year. Therefore preventing ovulation could be seen as a much easier target than blocking sperm production with every ejaculation. Men can produce a pretty much unlimited supply of sperm over the course of a year. So, it makes it extra challenging to finesse a product and dosage to curb that.

There are also issues around the role female partners play in the development of male contraception. Pregnancy is one of the most risky things a woman will do in her life, meaning the risks associated with contraception are almost always lower than the potential risks of pregnancy. For men, though, using contraception is different and it raises ethical questions. Given they obviously can't get pregnant, it's predominantly about preventing risk of 'harm' to another person, i.e. preventing pregnancy in their sexual partner. This means they'd be taking on the potential medical risks associated with hormonal contraception without directly experiencing the benefits. This is what's called 'shared risk' and it is an important aspect in the ethics of developing male contraceptives. It's the idea that exposing the man to a small risk in their contraception is worth it in order to prevent a much bigger risk occurring for the woman (i.e. unintended pregnancy).[16] This sense of dual responsibility is fundamental in developing male birth control.

The fact that couples need to be involved in trials can make a study more complex for scientists to run and to monitor results. Clinical research of this kind is also hugely expensive and, as we mentioned earlier in this chapter, it isn't easy to get the funding required.

## So, where have we got to?

We've mentioned (ranted) about this research a lot at The Lowdown. There was a clinical-phase study carried out years ago into the male contraceptive injection, which aimed to prevent pregnancy by reducing sperm count to below 'fertile' levels.[17] It began with 320 healthy men in heterosexual relationships. Every eight weeks, they were given the injection, containing synthetic testosterone and norethisterone enanthate (a progestogen), which would reduce their sperm count. As the trials progressed, the results looked promising, with efficacy similar to female methods. However, due to twenty participants experiencing negative side effects like mood swings, acne and libido changes (sound familiar?), and one case of depression, the trial ended early.

This was a breakthrough study, in that it showed real potential for creating a viable male method, so it's disappointing that it didn't progress further. It makes us wonder if the female hormonal methods created decades ago were being trialled today, would the side effects that so many of us experience prevent them advancing through clinical trials?

## What can we look forward to?

Gels, pills and the 'reversible vasectomy' appear to be our best bets for what we can expect to see first. The most common approach to developing male hormonal contraception centres around suppressing fertility by 'switching off' sperm production using testosterone and progestogen. This allows the body to continue to produce and ejaculate semen, but without sperm (or enough sperm) to be fertile and cause pregnancy. There's also research underway that explores whether heat can be used in the development of contraception to halt sperm production. Unlike female hormonal contraceptives which begin working quickly, within a week or even less, it can take a few months to curb sperm production. Non-hormonal methods focus around filtering out the sperm from the semen. Some of these don't require long-term commitment or involve the potential side effects that hormonal methods may bring.

Some of this research is decades in the making and studies continue to investigate their efficacy and the long-term impact. The hope is that the research provides enough conclusive results that scientists get the go-ahead to work with pharmaceutical companies to create products available for sale or prescription.

*Pre-clinical and early clinical trials*

- **COSO testicle ultrasound bath** This won the James Dyson award in 2021 for its clever design. It's a reversible male contraceptive that heats up testicles (stay with us) using ultrasound waves through water. Its creation is based on research that found ultrasound contraception has been successful on animals but it hasn't been tested on humans yet so it may be a way off.[18] It's a fascinating idea, though, and well worth googling to see how it works.
- **Thermal underwear or rings** These work by pushing the testicles up into the abdomen in order to heat them up a couple of degrees, which may halt sperm production.
- **Male non hormonal pill TDI-11861** In pre-clinical studies, TDI-11861 has been shown to temporarily immobilise

sperm in mice, preventing them from fertilising eggs for up to two and a half hours. The effects are reversible, with sperm regaining normal motility within twenty-four hours.[19]

*Phase 1*

- **Male non-hormonal pill YCT-529** This blocks a specific vitamin (vitamin A) pathway in the testes, which is necessary for making sperm. Studies have seen great results in animals, where it was effective in preventing pregnancies and was completely reversible once the treatment was stopped. Researchers have been studying this pill for a long time; in fact, blocking vitamin A to prevent sperm production was first discovered in the 1930s and the first human trials were conducted over sixty years ago.[20]

**Vasagel aka the reversible vasectomy**

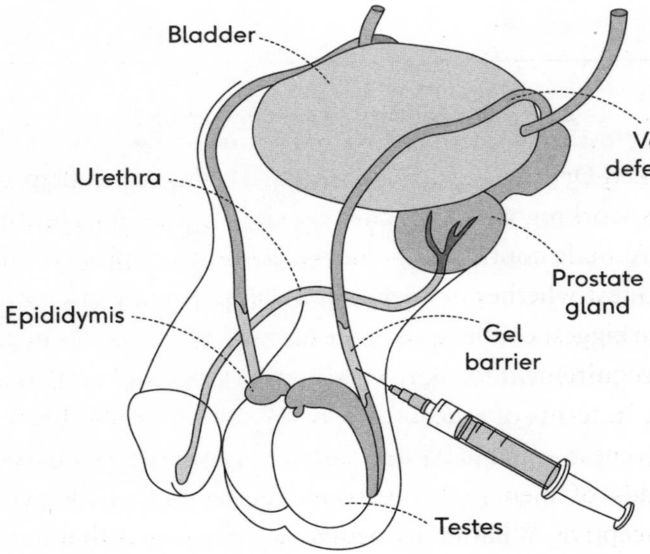

- **Smart RISUG (reversible inhibition of sperm under guidance)** Aka the 'reversible vasectomy', this is another reversible non-hormonal male contraceptive that could be a promising alternative. RISUG prevents pregnancy by injecting chemicals which partially block the vas deferens (the tube that transfers sperm) in order to deactivate sperm before they leave the body. It lasts about ten years and for anyone wishing to stop firing blanks during that time, another injection is administered to dissolve the contraceptive. Similar contraceptives are also being developed in the United States (Valsalgel or 'Plan A') and China.[21]
- **ADAM™** This is a similar long-acting reversible contraceptive that is being dubbed the IUD for men. It works by injecting a gel into the vas deferens. The gel blocks the sperm duct, stopping sperm from making it into semen. The procedure takes between twenty to thirty minutes and the gel lasts for about one year before the effects wear off.

**At home fertility tests for men?**

We asked Dr John Amory, an expert on male birth control who is working with the team developing the Valsalgel or 'Plan A' male contraceptive in the US how couples will be able to test whether new male contraceptives are effective.

'The biggest challenge in male contraceptive development is the requirement for both very high efficacy and very high safety. In terms of efficacy, my research shows that higher effectiveness – that is 95 per cent or 99 per cent – increases the odds of men in many countries trying a new male contraceptive. What many people don't realise is that male contraceptives that block sperm passage, such as Plan A, or approaches that block sperm production, will be very easy for men to monitor with at-home sperm check devices. This is different from female contraceptives and has the potential to improve men's and couples' confidence in their male contraceptives. Couples would simply need to buy a post-vasectomy or fertility test, that looks like a COVID test or pregnancy test, and have two lines which appear if sperm is detected in the semen sample.'

*Phase 2*

- **Male hormonal pills** Two oral contraceptives (DMAU and IIB-MNTDC) are being developed by the same team of researchers, and contain hormones that block sperm production. As with the female pill, this would be taken every day, and it would take sixty to ninety days of taking the pill to stop sperm being produced. If this continues in the right direction, it's thought that this may be available to the general public in the not too distant future.
- **Male contraceptive gel NEST/T** This gel containing testosterone and nestorone (a type of progesterone) is applied to the skin every day to the upper arms and shoulders. It works by acting on the signals from the brain to the testicles, which stimulate the testicles to make testosterone and sperm. The gel turns off that signalling pathway, so stops sperm and testosterone from being produced. Because men need testosterone to maintain their health, the gel also adds synthetic testosterone back into the body, but not enough to kick start sperm production. Trials have shown promising results and clinical research continues.

**What's it like to be on a male contraceptive trial?**

JJ and Heather are based in Edinburgh and have been together for six years. They were one of 400 couples worldwide to be selected for the NEST/T trial. Here JJ shares his experience of trialling a male contraceptive gel:

Q: Why did you both decide to take part in the trial?

**A:** Heather wasn't having a great time with contraception, and I recalled having read an article in the *Guardian* about male contraception being trialled in Edinburgh. I thought it might be a good way to relieve her of having to be the one feeling the effects of contraception for at least a while.

Q: What did it involve?

**A:** Monthly visits, physical examinations, producing sperm samples. The gel is applied daily to the shoulders and must stay on for a handful of hours, ideally all day or night. As it contains testosterone, you have to wear a top at all times until washing the gel off, to prevent it rubbing off on, for example, your partner.

Q: Did you have any side effects or impact on your relationship?

**A:** My testosterone levels initially dropped, which caused me to lose all emotional regulation skills – lots of crying. After that was sorted, there were no side effects or impact other than having to think about wearing a top most of the time. My routine was to put it on in the morning and wash it off in the evening, so I didn't have to wear a top to bed.

The most annoying part was having to plan sweat-inducing and water-based activities around the gel so it doesn't get washed off too soon after having been put on.

Many women seem quite scared to be able to trust a man to take contraception, but that wasn't our experience at all. My mum was famously terrible at taking contraception, which caused considerable stress in my parents' marriage, and Heather isn't great at it either! Putting on the gel at the same time as brushing your teeth in the morning felt very natural for me and I'm sure would easily become routine for other men too.

We don't know exactly when these or other male contraceptives will be made available to the public. There is still plenty of research to be done through rigorous clinical trials to ensure their safety and efficacy. As with female contraceptives, there need to be plenty of options out there for men to choose the method that suits their lifestyle and preferences. We're hopeful, though, that more male methods *will* become a reality. Watch this space!

## Female contraceptive developments

We all know that for contraception to be used effectively it needs to be easy to incorporate into life, with few (or preferably no) downsides. So, how can methods be improved?

Well, what is frustrating – but exciting too – is that there is so much we are still learning about how to not get pregnant. After the pioneering pill development in the 1950s and '60s, what the world should have witnessed was more leaps of progress. We should have seen scientists building on everything they were learning about reproductive health to explore other ways to prevent pregnancy – for women *and* men. What followed, though, was a research vacuum, a continuous feedback loop of rehashing the same techniques to the detriment of making further significant strides.

This leads to opportunities, though, which are happening *now*. Take genomics (i.e. the study of genes), which explores a totally different approach to stopping fertility in women and men. By targeting specific molecules in the body, scientists are researching whether it would be possible to switch off a man's sperm production and inhibit female ovulation.[22] We've barely dipped our toe in discovering other possible routes to stop unintended pregnancy and we need to see a much more dynamic approach.

## Improved and new contraceptive methods (now, please)

What are the other ways we might expect improvement on existing methods?

- **Timing** Lots of people find it inconvenient to take a pill at a similar time each day, or to make it to regular contraception appointments (e.g. for their injections). Research is currently underway with the hope of developing a pill that can be taken just once a month.[23] There is also research being carried out into a contraceptive injection that lasts six months which can be administered at home (a game changer for those who are not within easy access of a doctor's surgery or health clinic).[24]
- **Injection alternatives** Microarray patches (MAPs) are a relatively new technology that have primarily been used to deliver vaccinations as an alternative to needles. This has been particularly vital in countries where access to life-saving vaccines is difficult. Patches are much easier to administer (without medical experts, if necessary), pain-free and don't

leave hazardous waste in need of disposing.[25] Current research is underway to see how microarray patches could be utilised to deliver hormonal contraceptives.[26] A bit like the hormonal contraceptive patch, a plaster-like sticker which contains synthetic hormones is pressed onto the skin. You then remove the sticky plaster and the hormones are left to dissolve into the skin and work their contraceptive magic. There is no patch left on the skin, so it's very discreet.

- **Biodegradable implant** The Casea S implant is a long-acting method designed to release etonogestrel (a type of progestogen) into the body, which protects against pregnancy for eighteen to twenty-four months. Rather than needing a healthcare professional to remove it (as with the current implant), it would biodegrade. This may make it appeal more to those who struggle to access contraceptive care. If successful, it's thought that this will lessen the burden not just on individuals but on healthcare systems too.[27] At the time of writing, it's in Phase 1 trial stage.
- **Saheli** This is a non-hormonal contraceptive pill taken weekly. While traditional oral contraceptives contain oestrogen and progestogen or are progestogen-only, Saheli contains ormeloxifene, which is a non-steroidal oral contraceptive. The perks of this pill means it doesn't induce the side effects that many people experience on hormonal contraception. However, it is currently (at the time of writing) only available in India, due to licensing issues.
- **Mifepristone** This is an anti-hormonal drug and is one of the main medications used in medical abortions. Research is under way to explore whether it could be used as a flexible and mostly side-effect-free alternative to the pill. It works by blocking the pregnancy hormone progesterone and just like the emergency contraceptive pill, it delays ovulation. At the time of writing, a research study is investigating whether

mifepristone could be taken as a low-dose weekly pill that offers reliable contraception.[28] Researchers are also looking at whether it can be used as an emergency contraceptive pill. Watch this space for results!

As we've said, scientists haven't exactly reinvented the wheel with these new contraceptive offerings but all the same, it's exciting to hear about any progress. We look forward to collecting more data from Lowdown users who choose these methods.

# Conclusion

## from Alice, Founder & CEO of The Lowdown

So that's it. Pretty much everything you should need to know about how not to get pregnant, get pregnant and what happens when you stop being able to get pregnant. I hope that this book has given you a practical and balanced view of contraception and reproductive health, and will serve you as a companion that you can refer back to, no matter what age or life stage you are in. For now, I'd like to end with five key take-outs:

- **Don't suffer** Being on the wrong contraception for you can really impact your well-being – your mental health, your career, your relationships and your sex life. I know my story is extreme, but we should not have to put up with feeling emotional or unhappy because we don't want to get pregnant. Nor should we be unaware of some of the great benefits that contraception can offer, if we're suffering from painful periods or have a condition like PCOS or fibroids. Track your symptoms or side effects, take five minutes to book that GP appointment, and do some research. If you don't feel like you're getting the right advice or you're not being listened to, keep pushing and ask for a second opinion. It could make a huge difference to your day-to-day life and well-being.

- **It's a journey, and contraception is your co-pilot** Life would be boring if we didn't change. Something that we see time and time again is how our bodies and experiences transform over the decades; from our first period to our last. The chapters in this book around conditions, fertility, abortion, postpartum and menopause show how much of a gateway and partner your contraception is throughout and after your reproductive years. We've also shown how your body and needs can change; so if you have a negative experience, research your options and consider getting advice or trying something different.
- **You're the boss** One of the reasons I set up The Lowdown was that I noticed a paternalistic attitude to contraception from many healthcare professionals, and I wanted to change this by providing women with accurate, in-depth information so they can make informed decisions about what's best for them. As the chapter on health risk shows, these are complex and sometimes overwhelming areas that take a while to unpack. But that doesn't mean we should shy away from them, or assume women are not interested. In fact, when The Lowdown was born, some academics and medics were worried that reviews about contraceptives would be too negative and put women off using contraception completely ... but we've seen that women report both the negative and the positive, and are obviously intelligent enough to work out that side effects are individual and make their own informed choice.
- **It's not an even playing field** Health equality aims to treat everyone equally and in the same way. However, in healthcare, we recognise that health *equity* is far more important. Equity prioritises support and investment for groups who may have greater need. Sadly, women across the world, and

indeed within the UK, still have varying experiences with access to contraception and treatment of reproductive health, with many women in great need. The racial disparities faced by women with endometriosis are horrific; Black women are fifty times less likely to be diagnosed with endometriosis than white women, and their diagnosis takes on average two and a half years longer. And this is just one example of the inequality women of colour face. Not only that, but the gap between the least and most deprived areas in our country is stark. Healthy life expectancy (the age before someone is expected to develop a chronic illness or disability) is twenty years lower in poorer areas than richer ones ... and this is widening.[1] Three times more girls aged between thirteen and fifteen access emergency contraception in the poorest areas than the richest, due to lack of access to long-term contraception.[2] And women have a 65 per cent higher risk of getting cervical cancer in poorer areas than richer.[3]

If you're reading this book, you're already ahead, as you have access to a book, can read English to a very good level, and have the time and opportunity to read ... and if you think women's health isn't good enough, imagine what it's like for other women living in vulnerable or difficult circumstances? That is why we need to use our voices, to improve things not only for ourselves, but for all the women who may not have a voice. We know we keep banging on about it, but hopefully it's clear: we all need more investment in women's health and contraception, and we want to be involved.

- **Get involved and make your voice heard** The success of The Lowdown is testament to the power of women's voices, and how much they have been silenced. For centuries, our voices have not been heard, due to patriarchal nonsense, relentless underfunding and ignorance of women's health issues, and double standards in the way we are treated by society and the medical establishment. My belief is that healthcare is not always a two-way patient–doctor interaction; there's a huge amount of care and support that people get from sharing their experiences. That could be asking relatives about their experiences with hormones or menopause; talking to your friends during the years of childrearing about changes to your body and societal pressures, or talking with your mates if you're embracing your sexual freedom – whatever the context!

Every time someone shares their experience on The Lowdown, they help another person who is struggling in a similar situation. That's the truth. It may only be one other person; it's likely to be hundreds of people, as millions of women come to us for health information. The more women share through our platform, the more our data can be used as evidence that we need better healthcare for all women. We know a lot of platforms ask for your feedback for no good reason, but we will use it (with your consent) for positive social change. Through working with organisations like the NHS, and indeed writing this book, we're doing that. While medical research plays catch-up, we can help each other out and spread the knowledge we do have. Please share your experience at thelowdown.com and help us change the narrative around women's health.

# Appendix: Talking to your doctor

There are many factors that can impact a person's experience of healthcare, including ethnicity, religion or culture, sex and sexuality, gender identity, age, ability and socio-economic background. On page 358, we've included resources for further information and support on health equity.

Something that builds trust and confidence in seeking medical advice is feeling truly listened to. Being properly heard is one of the founding pillars of The Lowdown, and unfortunately it comes as little surprise that responses to the Women's Health Strategy survey of nearly 100,000 people confirms what we hear all too often: 84 per cent of respondents said that there have been instances where they didn't feel listened to by their healthcare professional.[1] Whatever area of your health you're seeking advice about, knowing how to advocate for yourself is hard.

We're caught in an unfortunate cycle that benefits no one. Healthcare professionals are under pressure to see more patients than ever but are receiving less funding, have fewer resources and less time. The average number of patients each full-time GP is responsible for is now 2,291 – an increase of 18 per cent per GP since 2015 – which is causing more instances of burnout in the profession.[2] These growing pressures lead to patients feeling dismissed, without answers and a growing mistrust in the medical system, despite your healthcare professional really trying their best in these challenging circumstances. We're here to be the middle(wo)man. Much of the info in this book is designed to arm you with everything you might need to know to help you get the best from your short time in the patient's chair.

Depending on where you live and the healthcare provision on offer, you may have a local practice whereby you can choose who you see, and in this practice, doctors may have different specialisms, such as a clinician with reproductive health expertise. In reality, that isn't the case for many, where waiting times are long and doctors are extremely stretched. How a GP or practice nurse can fit in a detailed consultation about reproductive health (or indeed many other things) in the allocated ten to fifteen minutes is a Herculean task. Even the very best doctors can struggle with this. Your GP really does want to help, and giving them as much info as you can will put you both in the best position. Here's how:

- **Keep a symptom diary** There are lots of reproductive conditions that benefit from symptom tracking. Keeping track of just about anything is helpful for doctors, especially when it comes to things like the level and type of pain you have, and other period symptoms. This could also include bowel symptoms, or skin, mood and energy levels. Basically, if you have a symptom that's bothering you, note it down and track it. If you prefer to do this digitally, there are lots of great tracking apps that make this easy (see Resources, page 358). Monitoring all of these symptoms will enable healthcare professionals to take a closer look at any patterns or irregularities in the short window you have with them, to help them get to the root of the cause.

- **Come prepared** Doctors usually have a limited window to see patients, so it helps to arrive at your appointment ready to clearly explain what's been going on and how you're feeling. As well as bringing your log of symptoms (see point above), it's good to know your medical history. Make a note of any questions you'd like to ask and, in turn, it can be helpful to take notes about what the doctor tells you.
- **Research** Whether you're unwell or suffering or are seeking a course of action (such as finding a contraceptive method to suit you), do your homework from trusted evidence-based sources (see Resources). If you notice yourself spending too much time going down a rabbit hole of self-diagnosis, then stop and take a breath. Don't panic, and remember that Google is not a doctor.
- **Bring someone** If seeing the doctor and/or explaining your symptoms, seeking medical information or making a request feels daunting, ask someone you trust to be there with you for support.
- **Don't give up** If needed, request to see a GP at the practice who is interested in contraception who may offer a fresh take. Or, go to a sexual health clinic or ask about women's health hubs in your area. You are not 'being difficult'. You know your body; trust your instinct when something doesn't feel right or if you sense that the advice/plan you receive from your doctor isn't quite hitting the mark.

## Your first contraception appointment

You may be a teen when you have your first contraception appointment or decades older. Whatever stage you're at, it's good to do some prep before attending. If you would feel more comfortable seeing a female doctor, then you're able to request that when you're booking your consultation. It's totally normal to feel a little apprehensive going to your first contraception appointment, whether that's at a GP surgery, pharmacy or a sexual health clinic. If you are a teenager or young adult, you might attend an appointment with a parent or guardian (though this is totally up to you).

If you're in the UK (and this will be similar in many other countries too), most GP appointments will last around ten to fifteen minutes, which isn't a lot of time. This is why coming prepared is a good idea, having done your research on the different types of pill and any other methods you might want to try. Try to bring any relevant information from your medical history or your family's medical history – it can be helpful to know if there are significant medical conditions that may run in your family, like a history of blood clots at a young age, for example. And make a list of any questions you may like to ask, or use our checklist.

**Questions to ask when choosing contraception**

- How effective is this method?
- How does it work?
- How long does it last?
- How regularly does it need to be taken/changed?
- Can I use this method with my medical history or family history?
- What side effects might I experience?
- How will it affect my periods?
- Are there any risks associated with this method?

- Will this type of contraception affect my weight/skin/moods, etc.?
- How and when do I start it?
- How soon after starting will I be protected from pregnancy?
- Are there any types of medication that may make it less effective?
- How soon after stopping the contraception could I get pregnant?

If you're a teenager, this appointment may feel like a step into the big, bad world of adulthood – embrace it! You're taking a leap in advocating for your well-being.

**Questions you may be asked by a healthcare professional**

- Why you're interested in taking contraception (i.e. for contraception, to manage periods or other conditions, or any other reason you may have). They're not asking this to be nosy or judgemental, but to help suggest the type of contraception they feel will suit you best.
- Whether you've taken another type of hormonal contraception before, or are taking any other medication.
- How your periods are (e.g. regular/irregular, heavy, painful, etc.).
- If you've recently had a baby or are breastfeeding, or have recently been pregnant or had an abortion.
- Any relevant medical conditions like migraines, or

whether you smoke, along with any family history. This will help them assess any risk factors that might affect your contraceptive choice (more on this in Chapter 6).

- Any relevant lifestyle consideration which may make certain contraceptives, including types of pill, more or less suitable. For example, if your job prevents you from taking your pill at a similar time each day, or if you want to be discreet about taking contraception.
- Whether you have a personal preference for one type of pill (or other contraceptive) over another.

Based on their assessment, they may give you a brief overview of the options and signpost you to further info if you need it. They should talk you through risks and common side effects, particularly in the first three months as your body adjusts to the hormones. At the end of the appointment, they may offer you a prescription, which you can choose to take to a pharmacy and collect right away or you may want to take some time to digest your options. You absolutely do not have to decide there and then what you'd like to do (or not do). Pause, let the info sink in and do some more research. If additional questions occur to you after your appointment, schedule a follow-up appointment or continue your research from trusted sources.

## Contraceptives in the teenage years

Contraception in general is safe for people under eighteen, though the same potential risks apply as for adults, which we cover in Chapter 6. If you're under sixteen, your healthcare professional will NOT need parental or guardian permission to prescribe you contraception if you are competent to make the decision yourself. They will encourage you to speak to a parent or guardian but they won't make you. You'll be afforded doctor–patient confidentiality just like adults, and you can feel free to talk openly about your reasons for seeking contraception, or to ask any questions or general advice. The only way your parent or guardian could find out from them is if they are concerned you're at risk from abuse or any other serious harm, in which case they would usually try to discuss this with you first.

You may have the type of relationship with your parent or guardian that is really open and communicative, meaning you might find it straightforward to talk to them about wanting to start using contraception. Perhaps, over the years, you've discussed some of the big topics of life, from periods and menstrual health to sex and consent, meaning raising contraception won't feel too tricky. Or it may be a little more complicated, especially if your reasons for wanting contraception are to avoid pregnancy, and let's face it, it can be difficult to start those first conversations with our parents about sex (particularly if they have never brought up the subject with you). If you would like to tell them you are thinking about starting contraception, or would like them to accompany you to your medical appointment, or if you have *already* started taking it and want to fill them in, it can feel daunting.

If you can, try to pick a time when you can talk freely without the pressure of either of you needing to be somewhere else. If you feel comfortable doing so, you can tell them the reasons behind this decision and how you're feeling about it all generally – this will also help to show them how considered you're being in your approach to this decision. It can also be a good opportunity to ask them any relevant questions about your family's medical history. Similarly, if you do start using contraception – or any medication, for that matter – they can look out for you if you start to experience any unpleasant side effects. Ideally, it won't be a single conversation that is so awkward it never gets mentioned again, but an ongoing exchange, where you can check back in with them and vice versa.

If your parents are not receptive to talking about this with you, that doesn't mean you're doing anything wrong by taking control of your reproductive health – quite the opposite. In an ideal world, you'll be supported to make a decision that works best for you. However, even if your parents/guardians aren't keen on the idea of contraception (or even discussing it), remember that you can still schedule an appointment with a healthcare professional and it will remain confidential and that you can be offered a prescription without parental consent. Hopefully you have friends or other trusted people in your life you can talk to or who could go with you to your appointment if you're feeling awkward or nervous.

# Resources

## General

The Lowdown (thelowdown.com/) provides information on every subject covered in this book, often in greater detail. We're based in the UK but also draw on evidence-based sources and studies from around the world. We take guidance from the following:

National Health Service (NHS): www.nhs.uk/
Faculty of Sexual and Reproductive Healthcare (FSRH): www.fsrh.org/home
Family Planning Association (FPA): www.fpa.org.uk
World Health Organization (WHO): www.who.int
National Institute for Health and Care Excellence (NICE): www.nice.org.uk/guidance
Patient UK: patient.info

## Menstrual health support

Wellbeing of Women: www.wellbeingofwomen.org.uk
Days for Girls: www.daysforgirls.org

Freedom4Girls: www.freedom4girls.co.uk
Bloody Good Period and Bloody Good Employers: www.bloodygoodperiod.com

## Health equity

Trans health: www.wpath.org
Cysters: cysters.org
Wellbeing of Women Health Collective: www.wellbeingofwomen.org.uk/what-we-do/campaigns/the-health-collective
Clap Back on the Contraceptive Patch campaign by Reproductive Justice Initiative: www.change.org/p/join-us-to-clap-back-on-the-contraceptive-patch and reprojusticeinitiative.org

## Tracking apps

Flo: flo.health
Clue: helloclue.com/
Natural Cycles: www.naturalcycles.com
Ovusense: www.ovusense.com/uk

## Your overall health

Managing your blood pressure at home: www.bhf.org.uk/informationsupport/support/manage-your-blood-pressure-at-home
Home blood pressure diary: bihsoc.org/wp-content/uploads/2017/09/Home_blood_pressure_diary.pdf
Stop smoking services: www.nhs.uk/better-health/quit-smoking

Body Mass Index (BMI) calculator: www.nhs.uk/health-assessment-tools/calculate-your-body-mass-index/calculate-bmi-for-adults
Weight management services: www.nhs.uk/better-health/lose-weight
Sexual health services: www.nhs.uk/service-search/sexual-health
The Migraine Trust: migrainetrust.org

## Contraception

The Lowdown Missed Pill Calculator: thelowdown.com/missed-pill
The Lowdown – How to switch your contraceptive: thelowdown.com/blog/how-to-switch-your-contraceptive
NHS emergency contraception services: www.nhs.uk/contraception/emergency-contraception
Fertility UK – Fertility awareness practitioners: www.fertilityuk.org

## Mental health

Find NHS talking therapies: www.nhs.uk/mental-health/talking-therapies-medicine-treatments/talking-therapies-and-counselling/nhs-talking-therapies
MIND: www.mind.org.uk
Samaritans: available 24/7 365 days a year on 116 123
Shout text service available 24/7 365 days a year on 85258
Headspace app: www.headspace.com
Calm app: www.calm.com
Sleepio: www.sleepio.com

## PMDD

PMS and PMDD: www.pms.org.uk
International Association for PMDD: iapmd.org
Me v PMDD app (created by IAPMD): mevpmdd.com

## Endometriosis

Endometriosis UK: www.endometriosis-uk.org
The Endometriosis Foundation: www.theendometriosisfoundation.org

## Polycystic Ovary Syndrome (PCOS)

Verity PCOS: www.verity-pcos.org.uk
AskPCOS: www.askpcos.org

## Fibroids

British Fibroid Trust: www.britishfibroidtrust.org.uk
Fibroid Network: www.fibroid.network

## Abortion

Abortion Talk Helpline: www.abortiontalk.com 03330909266
The British Pregnancy Advisory Service: www.bpas.org
MSI Reproductive Choices: www.msichoices.org.uk/support
National Unplanned Pregnancy Advisory Service: www.nupas.co.uk

## Fertility

The Fertility Network UK: fertilitynetworkuk.org
British Fertility Society: www.britishfertilitysociety.org.uk/public-resources
HFEA: UK Fertility regulator: www.hfea.gov.uk
Adoption UK: www.adoptionuk.org
Gov.uk Foster Carer Guide: educationhub.blog.gov.uk/2022/11/10/everything-you-need-to-know-about-becoming-a-foster-parent
Find a fostering agency: www.nafp.org.uk/pages/7-find-a-fostering-agency
Surrogacy UK: surrogacyuk.org
Brilliant Beginnings Surrogacy Agency: brilliantbeginnings.co.uk

## Pregnancy

Preconception advice: www.nhs.uk/pregnancy/trying-for-a-baby/planning-your-pregnancy
Keeping healthy during pregnancy: www.nhs.uk/pregnancy/keeping-well
Use of medicines in pregnancy: www.medicinesinpregnancy.org
Antenatal Results & Choices: www.arc-uk.org

## Pregnancy loss

Tommy's charity: www.tommys.org/about-us
The Miscarriage Association: www.miscarriageassociation.org.uk

## Postnatal care

Breastfeeding helpline: 0300 100 0212 www.nationalbreastfeedinghelpline.org.uk
The Breastfeeding Network: www.breastfeedingnetwork.org.uk
Medicines while breastfeeding: www.breastfeedingnetwork.org.uk/drugs-factsheets
La Leche League breastfeeding support: laleche.org.uk
Pre- and post-natal depression awareness and support: pandasfoundation.org.uk
MummyMOT postnatal physio care: www.themummymot.com

## Perimenopause and Menopause

The Lowdown perimenopause symptom checker: www.thelowdown.com/blog/perimenopause-symptom-checker
Menopause Support UK: menopausesupport.co.uk
Rock My Menopause: rockmymenopause.com
Women's Health Concern: www.womens-health-concern.org

## Research

Finding out about research studies and getting involved:
www.isrctn.com
bepartofresearch.nihr.ac.uk
exeltis.com/entwine
thelowdown.com/blog/research
Male Contraceptive Initiative: www.malecontraceptive.org

# References

A lot of research has gone into writing this book, and many sources of reference have been examined. These sources are acknowledged with a number in the relevant position in the text. In order to save paper and keep the book to a manageable size, the corresponding details of these studies and surveys can be found on our website, using the QR code below.

# Thank yous

## From Alice

First and foremost, I want to say a huge thank you to all the women who have shared their experiences at The Lowdown, spread the word about our platform, or been a part of our journey. Since launching our website, the response has been overwhelming. Hearing how much we've helped you never gets old, and your messages and feedback continue to inspire me. A special thank you to those who agreed to have their experiences published in this book and to everyone who has participated in our surveys and research projects.

To Dr Mel and Dr Fran, my incredible co-writers – working with you both over the last five years has been an absolute privilege. I've learned so much from you about medicine, research and women's health. Thank you for your patience, dedication and tireless work in writing and reviewing countless edits. Your commitment to this project, as with everything you do, has been extraordinary.

Thank you to Georgia Gallant, our Content & Social Manager, for your invaluable help in writing this book and for creating so much of the content that has shaped our brand. To Dani Conlon, our Community & Partnerships Lead, for her incredible work engaging with our community of women and ensuring we had permission to share their experiences in this book. To our designer, Emma Wright, for her meticulous work in bringing this book to life with beautiful designs. And to John Fisher, Ellie Jones and Monique Devaux for their keen eyes in analysing our data, proofreading and checking references.

To the wider Lowdown team, past and present – thank you. Marija Ziterbart, our CTO, and her team of developers, for continuously building and improving our platform. Annie Coleridge, who expertly ran the company while I took time out to have my first son. And the many others, like Jen Penaluna, who have contributed their hard work along the way. A special thanks to our in-house medical experts – Dr Becky Mawson, Dr Nikki Ramskill and Dr Zaakira Mahomed – for their valuable insights, research and contributions to this book and their dedication to improving women's health.

I also wanted to say thank you to our friends at the Faculty of Sexual and Reproductive Health (FSRH), the Primary Care Women's Health Forum (PCWHF) and all the healthcare professionals who have contributed to our content, resources and tools. Collaborating with you has been an honour, and your guidance has been invaluable. A special thanks to Lindsay Thomas for her thorough review and feedback on this book, and to all the medical experts and researchers who have shared their knowledge and insights in this text.

Finally, to my family – my husband, Keiran, and my friends, Amber and Rose – thank you. Building The Lowdown has been anything but easy, and you've been there through the fundraises, legal disputes and the seemingly endless ups and downs of the past six years. And to my mum – I'm sorry I was such a hormonal and difficult teenager, but look at what came out of it! It was all worth it.

# Index